HARD CHOICES

ALSO BY B. D. COLEN

Take Care: Patients' Guide to Personal Health

The Family Medical Diary

Born at Risk: The Dramatic True Story of 24 Hours in an Intensive Care Nursery

Karen Ann Quinlan: Dying in the Age of Eternal Life

HARD CHOICES

Mixed Blessings of
Modern Medical Technology

B. D. COLEN

Foreword by John W. Scanlon, M.D.

G. P. PUTNAM'S SONS / NEW YORK

G. P. Putnam's Sons
Publishers Since 1838
200 Madison Avenue
New York, NY 10016

Portions of chapters 7, 8 and 14 appeared in different form in
Newsday. Material used with permission.

Library of Congress Cataloging-in-Publication Data

Colen, B. D.
  Hard choices.
  Includes index.
  1. Medical ethics.   I. Title. [DNLM: 1. Bioethics.
2. Economics, Medical.   3. Ethics, Medical.
4. Technology Assessment, Biomedical.   W 50 C692h]
R724.C547   1986   174'.2   85-30102
ISBN 399-13139-6

Printed in the United States of America
1   2   3   4   5   6   7   8   9   10

For my father, with love

AUTHOR'S NOTE

The persons whose personal hard choices you will read about in the odd-numbered chapters chose to be interviewed in the belief that making their private agonies public might help others facing similar dilemmas. Except for the couples in chapters 3 and 7, and the Hannans in chapter 5, who were willing to share their experiences but asked that their privacy be protected, real names and titles of individuals are used throughout the book. I hope that those who were willing to open up their lives to me, and to you, in this manner will feel that the effort was worthwhile.

B. D. Colen
Northport, New York
October 1985

Contents

CONTENTS

Foreword

A military arms instructor once remarked that the ideal weapon is not one that simply kills. Rather, it is one that maims, especially when the wounds are particularly disabling and gruesome. He said that the effect from such an "ideal" weapon requires more personnel, more services and more resources than a merely lethal one. Additionally, he argued that the very nature of the wounds demoralized those still whole and robbed them of their will to fight, their competitive urge. In a sense, modern technological medicine has created the social equivalent of a perfect weapon. Today, many a catastrophic illness visibly wounds the patient as it rages to consume accumulated resources and slowly demoralize the patient's loved ones. We are all potential targets, but the very young and the very old are most vulnerable. Consider, for example, the following two examples:

Her tired, sallow face was drawn into a perpetually agonized grimace, which was accentuated by each rasping breath. Gnarled hands picked restlessly at the thin sheet covering her emaciated body. Pain seemed the only stimulus able to reach the tattered remnants of her once vivacious consciousness. Sophisticated electronic devices had clearly documented permanent, serious brain damage. Changing her position, trying to bathe her, even attempting to feed her only elicited struggling, twisting, combative behavior. Oxygen whistled from holes in plastic tubes fixed in her nostrils. These tubes were relentlessly eroding her upper lip. The restraints on her arms had turned her parchmentlike skin into an endless opportunity for bacterial growth. Urine dribbling from her bladder catheter was a constant, blood-tinged reminder that she was unable to control even the most basic of body functions. No such reminder was needed for her family, whose daily visits went unrecognized. She was a woman in limbo, too sick to be in a nursing home, yet not sufficiently ill for the hospital's intensive care unit. A series of small strokes, an overwhelming bacterial infection "successfully" treated, chronically inadequate nutrition plus side effects from the pharmacopoeia of drugs used to treat the modern therapeutic daisy chain of problem-followed-by-complication had rendered her existence marginal, vegetative and incredibly expensive. She would die, of course, but not without several more weeks of medical heroics, family crises and financial loss. Her status implied a litany of unanswerable questions.

When her heart stops should she be resuscitated? If so, for how long? If her kidneys fail should she receive dialysis? Is she eligible to participate in any experimental studies? How valid or informed were any consents obtained from her family? If her insurance coverage runs out should she be transferred to a charity facility? Must her worldly goods be sold to cover hospital costs? How financially responsible are her children? What's the definition of death?

At the other extreme of life's spectrum lay a tiny, prematurely born baby boy. Though he weighed less than two pounds at birth, every organ was still functioning as if in its previous placenta-dependent fetal existence. These organs would not work in our world without great help. Most dramatically, his lungs filled with air poorly and required repeated mechanical in-

10

flation. The oxygen in his blood was insufficient to supply the acute needs of his body's cells, which kept forming toxic acids. These, in turn, produced further biochemical insult. His heart could not sustain this added burden for very long, and his immature nervous system was inadequate in basic control of the breathing and heart activity necessary to sustain existence outside the womb. Indeed, his brain was still in the process of developing its own anatomical structures, including those cellular contacts that appropriately network nervous impulses. His central nervous system was extraordinarily vulnerable to the slightest stress. A huge blood clot had already formed in those fluid-filled cavities that lie deep below the cortex of the intelligence-giving portion of the brain. And there was clear evidence that blood had already seeped into the brain's tissue, killing even more neurons.

He was attached by sensors to sophisticated electronic devices that monitored his breathing, heart function, blood pressure and the content of oxygen and carbon dioxide in his blood. Skilled nurses attended him constantly. Powerful medications and complex nutritional substances flowed into his blood through multiple intravenous lines. Frequent laboratory tests evaluated his body's chemistry, using tiny samples of blood and urine. This information was needed to manipulate prescriptions for intravenous fluids and their components in order to keep his bodily needs in balance and to permit growth even while he lay comatose.

There was the overwhelming probability that this tiny life, if it continued at all, would be lived terribly handicapped. He would walk alone, speak few words and think not at all. It was likely he would never ever feel love nor return it. Those who loved him, and visited daily or more frequently, had no way of knowing if he was aware of their visits or even if he found any solace in their touch. They were, however, fully aware of his bleak prognosis and that the meter was running at a rate of a thousand or more dollars a day. Their despair was tangible.

Those same tough questions about how much care for how long, whether experimentation is justified, and how vigorously to pursue financial recovery are appropriately asked in this circumstance, too. Attempts at answers are surprisingly complex, as we will see.

Both the parents of a sick newborn and the children of a dying parent are caught in a vortex of conflicting, often extraordinary feelings. To love is, among other things, to be able to sacrifice, to provide care and to do what's right and best for your loved one under the most trying circumstances. But what is right in the two situations above? What motives might underlie any decisions about care? Is euthanasia a consideration? If so, would choosing this option be governed by economic considerations as well as by the plight of the victim? Is anything less than doing everything conceivable a form of euthanasia? Who should make such hard choices? Is this role only for those who care and are legally empowered? What is the proper function of the physician? What help is available from society? What is legally or morally correct? Are they the same thing?

American society has taken a long, hard and broad look at modern medicine and discovered there are, indeed, very real limits to what can or should be done in many areas of medical care. Resource allocation, cost containment and "considering the big picture" have become buzzwords today. The gross national product is dominated by the health care industry. There is a massive drain on federal, state and local tax dollars for health care. Private insurance companies are screeching about escalating costs. They desire to cut benefits to the bone. Yet we all are enthralled when the Jarvik-7 gets sewn into another debilitated chest or when a baboon is sacrificed to give an imperiled new life a few more days of artificially sustained existence. Resources for these procedures come from the same monetary pie, although the piece of origin may not be immediately recognizable. They are all health care dollars and will eventually be paid by the tax-payer/subscriber. What about the California lady whose most prominent side effect from a common fertility drug was to bear seven very premature babies all at once? Who will ultimately pay for this medical misfortune?

There is another side here, seemingly a paradox that borders on hypocrisy. Although society (which is you and me) decries rising health care costs, when the crunch of serious illness comes to us, or to our loved ones, cheap alternatives are regularly discarded. We want our own doctor, not today's rotator at the HMO. We want a Jarvik-7, not solace and a compassionate death. We want, once again, what's right, what's best, and damn the cost. This issue is further confounded because the money for medical bills doesn't come directly from our own pocket. We don't have to peel a wad of bills from our wallet. Rather, payment is sent from the third-party carrier directly to the hospital and doctor. We just receive a neat computer printout with incomprehensible line items and indecipherable codes. We might fall off our chairs when the bottom line, after insurance payment, leaves a breath-taking balance that we must pay. But most of the time, money flows well beyond our appreciation. As such, the whole deal takes on the aura of unreality.

What about the emotional resources consumed? It is no accident that marriages dissolve with amazing frequency in families of handicapped newborns after the child is discharged from the intensive care nursery. Such dissolutions do not just take the form of divorce; suicide, alcoholism and spouse disappearances occur as well. Indeed, those agencies responsible for monitoring the quality of care in newborn intensive care facilities mandate that each hospital with such a unit must provide adequate psycho-emotional support systems for all parents. These supports include social workers, psychiatric consultative availability and discharge planning for parents of afflicted infants. The need is apparent, but who pays for these services? The costs are generally "absorbed" by the hospital into the daily bed rate and then spread among all patients. You can guess which services will be the first to go when real cost containment finally arrives.

It is also no accident that acts of violence against old people have escalated during the past several years. Reports of horrendous neglect, harassment, physical abuse, even homicide against the elderly by their relatives seem to appear daily in our newspapers. The sick senior citizen is, clearly, a reminder of our own mortal selves. He or she is also a reminder that physical dependency drains the provider emotionally as well as financially. The dependent patient loses self-esteem too, which further enhances his or her vulnerability as victim. Where does such rampant emotional disequilibrium impact when hard choices must be made for the dying elderly?

There is another participant to consider, too. In the striving for technological medical perfection, the "rescue all life at any cost" fantasy has profoundly affected today's medical practitioner.

For starters, legal consequences from critical-care decisions are constantly scrutinized both within and outside the hospital. There are possible criminal complaints to be answered if a willful act of euthanasia is performed. There is a constant assault on the clinical decision-making processes from many quarters. The recent, and ongoing, babies Doe debacle is a particularly unfortunate case in point. Here, a meddlesome federal government encouraged any concerned informant to call a toll-free hotline phone with suspicions about abuse or withdrawal of "appropriate" newborn care. During the hotline's trial, before the proposed regulations were overthrown on a legal technicality, more than four hundred phone calls were recorded. As expected, these ran the gamut from crank to ludicrous. Investigations into a few real tragedies revealed only that good, compassionate care was being given. But federal intrusion upset the hospitals and parents under investigation. Responsibility for such troubleshooting has now been relegated to local or state governments with federal oversight only implied. But, again, there is no clear definition of the clinical specifics upon which right and wrong decisions are judged. Sight seems to have been lost once again of the fact that government can't legislate ethics and morality. Those must come from within individuals.

The most malignant legal specter that looms over any physician's practice today is the threat of medical malpractice. That we who live in a country with the highest-quality medical care in the world also have the highest rate of medical malpractice seems a tribute mostly to the tenacity, perseverance, hard work and profit motive of the legal profession. Malpractice costs the public every time they visit a doctor, go to the hospital or pay a health insurance premium. The loss is not only in dollars. Trust and compassion get short shrift, too. Today, new patients are often regarded as potential litigants. Those extra tests ordered to "cover all bases," the reluctance to make a decision that stops heroic but hopeless care, or that detailed description about every possible horrible complication from necessary therapy, can be laid directly to the physician's fear of a subsequent malpractice action. Certainly the public needs protection from incompetent, bumbling, thoughtless or just plain stupid medical practice. And make no mistake, lousy care does exist. But it is not prevalent. Certainly it's not nearly as frequent as published figures about suits and their ultimate judgments would suggest. One out of every two American doctors will be sued sometime during his or her career. In some medical specialties, in certain geographical areas, malpractice insurance premiums will exceed $70,000 per doctor this year. Talk about gobbling up resources. Talk about making a soldier weary of the fray. Talk about demoralization. The ideal weapon strikes again.

Where do the medical schools stand in all of this? Centers of technological excellence in medicine are largely clustered in those hospitals intimately associated with accredited American medical schools. Surely, teaching the societal relevance of medical care is quite obviously the responsibility of medical educators. In my opinion, this has been inadequately done.

It is an interesting yet tragic fact that those people in most need of high-tech, crisis-oriented medical care have the least political, social or economic clout. Newborns don't vote and don't write to their congressmen. Their parents are episodic users of the intensive care facility. Once their own crisis has run its course, parents become too busy raising their child and taking him or her for multiple specialist physician visits to become politically active. Such parents are very frequently from lower-middle-class or poverty-level populations. Or else they are so new to the work force that they have little economic impact in the marketplace. It is no accident that supplies or drugs for the neonatal intensive care unit are difficult to obtain in sizes or strengths appropriate for the wide range in weights and ages of tiny patients.

At the other extreme of life, despite commendable consciousness-raising efforts by the Gray Panthers, the geriatric patient is not a very potent economic and political force. If your voice isn't heard, you don't get counted.

B. D. Colen is about to take you through the thorny wilderness that makes up the frontier of modern medical technology. He will discuss the great effort expended in keeping this frontier together and progressing. It is a sobering tour. It is all too easy to become preachy or morally indignant about how this or that could be allowed to happen. The reader is advised to remember that medicine is practiced by humans on humans. Each participant brings a set of personal biases, ethics and emotional hang-ups to each crisis circumstance. There may well be hidden agendas as well as multiple, subtle pressures on the part of all participants to achieve a certain outcome. But remember, in the context of critical-care medicine, decisions *must* always be made. It is my view that physicians and responsible adults involved in these life-and-death situations are the only ones who will ever be in an appropriate position to make the really hard choices. They will always need help and support, as well as social, legal and governmental institutions sufficiently flexible to allow individualization in each case. These players will always need compassion and emotional peace, never anger or bureaucratic red tape. This simple notion should form the basis for the hard choices society must soon make.

JOHN W. SCANLON, M.D.
Professor of Pediatrics, Georgetown University School of Medicine
Chief of Neonatology, Columbia Hospital for Women

Introduction

It was a glorious Sunday afternoon in late October 1973. The breeze was barely strong enough to break up the mirrorlike surface of the Chesapeake Bay, but that didn't seem to bother us as we gently bobbed beside the Thomas Point light. I was stretched out on the port side of the cockpit, with my right leg draped haphazardly over the tiller. I wasn't paying much attention to other boats that might be drifting toward us, but it was late enough in the season for us to have most of the bay to ourselves. If I was concentrating on anything at all it was on not being lulled to sleep, when I thought I heard my sister-in-law say something about "pulling the plug."

"Pulling what?" I sat up.

"Pulling the plug. Shutting off respirators. You know," replied Sue. No, I really didn't know. I was then a general assignment reporter on the Metropolitan staff of the *Washington Post* and knew nothing more about respirators or "pulling the plug" than did any other layman—which, a year and a half before the case of Karen Ann Quinlan, meant that I knew next to nothing.

"You mean they're pulling plugs in the unit?" I asked Sue, who worked as a nurse at the Maryland Institute for Emergency Medicine—the shock trauma unit—in Baltimore.

"Of course they pull plugs," said Sue, exasperated at my naïveté. "That's not the problem."

"What is the problem then?"

"The nurses are all getting upset because they're pulling the plugs too soon."

"Too soon? What's too soon?"

"Oh, when they get a 'high quad' from a motorcycle accident or something like that, they're only waiting about ten days or so and then they shut them off," she told me. And that was enough, enough to intrigue me, and my editors at the *Post*, and enough to start me down the road toward a series of articles entitled "A Time to Die," which began running in the *Post* on March 10, 1974, one year and forty-five days before Karen Ann Quinlan became comatose. The first article began:

About four times in the past year, doctors at the Maryland Institute for Emergency Medicine turned off the respirator that was maintaining the life of a quadriplegic patient whose body was completely and irrevocably paralyzed—but whose brain was functioning.

Each time the institute receives such a patient, it keeps the person alive for a few weeks, long enough to determine if the patient's condition will improve to the point where he can again lead a meaningful life. And each time the doctors end up turning off the respirator.

The quadriplegics are never told their respirators are going to be turned off, and their families are told only obliquely, according to Dr. William Gill, clinical director of the institute. Gill said the unit receives about four such patients a year.

However, said Gill, the respirator is never turned off if a family asks that it remain on.

"It's illegal, I suppose some people would argue that," said Gill. "[But] you're not actively doing anything to worsen the patient's state according to what the patient's state was when he came in here. All you are doing is using artificial support to see if you can

19

do something [to save the patient] and then withdrawing that support when we find there is nothing we can do.

"We use that as a rationalization in our own mind," said Gill.

Apparently the rationalization was a good one. There were no suits, no charges, no formal investigations of the procedures in the unit, despite the publicity. Instead, the articles on what were then the practices in the shock trauma unit—I am told they have changed considerably in the years since then—and about the withdrawal of care from premature and sick babies caused a brief flurry of letters and telephone calls to the *Post,* and that was that. Then a twenty-one-year-old New Jersey woman named Karen Ann Quinlan apparently had too much to drink while celebrating a friend's birthday, passed out on her bed and never woke up. We will never know precisely what caused Quinlan's coma, although the best medical speculation is that she vomited, aspirated the vomit and blocked off her oxygen supply long enough to leave her in a chronic vegetative state.

But whatever caused the brain damage, the case of "the girl in the coma" made issues surrounding the care of the dying and terminally ill a subject of national debate for more than a decade. When Quinlan's parents went into Superior Court in Morristown, New Jersey, and filed a petition asking that Joseph Quinlan be named his daughter's guardian for the express purpose of ordering the removal of the respirator thought to be sustaining her life, literally hundreds of journalists from around the world poured into the quiet county seat for the two-week hearing. Pictures of Karen Ann Quinlan became a staple of the evening television news and the front pages of newspapers as her parents pleaded that she be allowed to die a "natural death" should that be "God's will."

Quinlan's death was neither God's will nor that of Superior Court Judge Robert Muir, who refused the family's request. But the following March the New Jersey Supreme Court made history when it reversed Muir and granted to the incompetent through their representatives the same right to refuse treatment long held by competent patients. So Quinlan's respirator was finally removed. But not only did she not die when the respirator was turned off, she did not die for another nine years. It was not until June 11, 1985, that the body of Karen Ann Quinlan finally gave out. And for those intervening nine years, her father continued to visit her bedside twice a day, and both her parents became active in the hospice movement, which had hardly begun in this country at the time Karen became comatose.

While the case of Karen Ann Quinlan involved only the rights and care of the dying, it raised our national consciousness and made it possible for us to at least consider a whole host of bioethical issues, some of which faced us a decade ago and some of which arose afterward. Ironically, while we are now able to discuss those issues, and while a Quinlan-like case causes barely a media ripple today, we are not much closer to solving any of these difficult problems than we were when I wrote my series for the *Washington Post*. In fact, there are those such as Daniel Callahan, director of the Hastings Center, who would argue it is more difficult for a physician to turn off a respirator today than it was a decade ago, in part because of the current climate of malpractice litigation and in part for the very reason that we *do* discuss these issues today. Because everyone is now aware that "plugs" are pulled, that care is withdrawn, some physicians have become more leery of taking such action, believing that they may become the victims of overzealous prosecutors or the objects of suits brought by distraught relatives.

But the problems surrounding the care of hopelessly ill adults represent only a small portion of the issues dealt with in this book. And arriving at answers to most of these questions requires that we put a price tag on human life.

INTRODUCTION

There are some who will find crass the suggestion that we consider the value of human life in terms of dollars. They are right,
of course. But they are also naïve, for we in this country have always been willing to equate dollars and life, even if we are squea-
mish about admitting that we do so. For example, one hundred
and twenty-five years ago we fought the Civil War over the pre-
cise dollar value of human life: Southerners argued that blacks
were simply property, and extremely valuable property at that,
while Northerners, whose economic system did not depend upon
slave labor, argued that, while certainly not equal to whites,
blacks at least ought to be freed from slavery. And in our own
day, we do little to improve coal mine safety, thus condemning
miners to death, simply because making the mines really safe
would be so expensive as to raise the price of coal. Thus, we put a
price on the value of a miner's life. We continue to subsidize the
tobacco industry because of the economic implications of not
doing so, and yet by supporting tobacco farmers we place a price
on the lives of those who will die of lung cancer and smoking-
related heart disease.

Granted, money is not central to all the hard choices addressed
in this book. Whether or not we should proceed toward somatic,
or germ cell, gene therapy, for example, involves ethical and biological questions rather than monetary ones. Genetic research is
not inexpensive, but money is not the key issue here. Rather, the
issue is whether we want to attempt to correct genetic defects in
affected individuals but have them pass the defect on to future
generations, or whether we want to remove the defect from the
genetic line and take the risks that such genetic manipulation can
entail.

And when we speak of fetal therapy—which is also expensive—the real issue is not the cost but what we say about the
rights and value of the fetuses we treat, and thus all fetuses. Can
our society long tolerate the moral schizophrenia that calls a

22

fetus a patient on one floor of a hospital while that same fetus is a "thing" devoid of all rights and humanity, fair game for extinction, on another floor? Here the questions are strictly ethical, or moral or religious, rather than financial. Obviously some women, and couples, opt for abortion in response to what may be horrendous financial pressures, but eliminating such pressures would not eliminate the need for, and debate over, abortion.

When we move on, however, to discussions of new reproductive methods, money becomes an important issue. Ethical and legal questions are still significant here in and of themselves: What rights does a frozen embryo have? Who has the right to a child when a surrogate mother refuses to give it up as promised? Do surrogate arrangements, or in vitro fertilization, threaten the family as we know it? At the same time, we have to begin to consider finances when we speak of the "new conceptions": Should medical insurance cover infertility treatment? Should the government, in an age of ever-increasing worldwide overpopulation, finance research to improve couples' chances of bearing children? Should private venture capitalists be financing scientific research, and if they should, should certain medical technologies, such as embryo transfer, be available only to the rich or those willing to make enormous sacrifice to pay for them?

As we discuss the issues surrounding neonatal care, money becomes an ever-larger consideration in assessing the hard choices we must make. We are now spending upward of $2 billion a year in this country to care for premature and sick infants, most of whom would have died had they been born two decades ago. Is this money well spent? Do we really want to be expending our resources saving pound-and-a-half babies in an era when we are cutting back on childhood immunization and school lunch programs? Should we be spending an average of $140,000 per baby for neonatal intensive care when about 15 percent of the survivors suffer from defects of one sort or another? These are easy questions to duck. They are not easy questions to answer.

And what of the babies Doe, those severely handicapped infants whom the Reagan administration would force physicians and parents to save at all costs. Would saving a baby with Down's syndrome or spina bifida or any one of a number of major birth defects really be an issue if money were freely spent on the care of handicapped children and adults? Would parents opt to have their baby die from lack of medical treatment, or feeding, for that matter, if they knew that they could depend upon the government to help them care for a handicapped child? Wouldn't most parents rather go through life knowing that they had placed a handicapped infant in a humane, safe, caring institution than knowing that they had opted for the death of the child? But there are few, if any, such institutions, and the same administration that is pushing so hard to save these babies has been cutting off funds to help pay for their care. So here we are clearly putting a price on life.

Should we be paying a quarter of a million dollars each for liver transplants that, at best, succeed only about two-thirds of the time? And if we decide to have private insurance and public insurance programs pay for liver transplants for children, can we deny those same transplants, and payments, to fifty-five-year-old alcoholics with cirrhosis? Is it right that we have a system that essentially requires that those in need of transplants hold community bake sales and car washes to pay for the potentially life-sustaining operation? And who gets the organs that are available? How do we decide, with a limited supply of organs, who shall live and who shall die?

If organ transplants present us with difficult questions, the questions posed by artificial organ programs are mind-boggling. We take kidney dialysis for granted now, but we never stop to think about the fact that we are spending $2 billion a year on dialysis for only about 60,000 people. Many of these patients lead normal, productive lives, but many do not. At least one study showed that dialysis patients have a suicide rate four hundred times the national average. And many patients lead bleak, depressing lives dependent upon their thrice-weekly visit to the dialysis center. By way of contrast, just think for a minute of what even a single year's worth of that money could do to relieve famine in the drought-plagued areas of Africa, or what $2 billion a year could do to bring job training programs or mass transportation to our central cities. Should we really be spending that money on maintaining the lives of 60,000 chronically ill patients, or should we be using it to save literally millions of lives in Africa or to reshape our urban socio-economic landscape?

The financial, medical and ethical difficulties we have encountered in the artificial kidney program are only the tiniest foretaste of what is to come from a program to provide artificial hearts to all who need them. Estimates are that such a program could cost as much as $40 billion per year. What will we give up to fund that? Neonatal care? Corrective heart surgery for children? And what quality of life will we be buying with those billions of dollars, the quality of life provided to Barney Clark and William Schroeder?

All of which brings us back to Karen Ann Quinlan and the questions we face for ourselves and our loved ones in approaching the end of life. How much of our health care dollar do we want to expend on the dying process? Are we satisfied with the present allocation of resources, which has us spending the greatest proportion of Medicare funds on those in the last six months of life? Is it right that we spend more to go into the hospital to die than we do to go into the hospital and recover? Do we really want to spend more than $120,000 to keep a dying patient alive for a few more months?

What price, then, do we want to put on life? What must be the

25

quality of the life we preserve and extend? These are questions most of us would rather not ask, much less attempt to answer. But these questions are now being asked indirectly when the federal budget moves through the Office of Management and Budget each year, and are answered on a strictly political, or emotional, basis, with no thought given to their long-term ethical implications. If we don't face up to these hard choices now, and give them serious thought, we will wake up in a few short years and find that the questions we never asked were answered—in ways that we may not like at all.

I.
THE GENETIC THREAD

CHAPTER 1

The Short Life of Justin Micha Fleisher

There is a special bogeyman who haunts the dreams of some new mothers, particularly first-time mothers. He comes in many different forms and is known by many names—SIDS (sudden infant death syndrome), meningitis, drowning, leukemia, brain tumor—but whatever he is called, his threat is the same: He will take the life of the infant sleeping in the crib nearby.

Ellen Fleisher's bogeyman didn't have a name, at least not at first. All she knew was that he would claim the life of Justin Micha Fleisher, her first-born. "I just had this mother's intuition that he wasn't going to live very long . . . from the time he was born I just had a terrible feeling that that little boy was never going to grow up." Jeff Fleisher would find his wife standing beside Justin's crib in the middle of the night, sobbing in the dark in the room with the bright yellow walls decorated with pictures of ducks and raccoons and Winnie the Pooh. In the days after Justin and Ellen returned from Fairfax (Virginia) hospital, Ellen began to "pick him up out of his sound sleep and just sit in the bentwood rocker and sob with this child in my arms. I just knew he was going to die and I wanted to hold him as much as I could."

As she sat holding her infant, Ellen would pray for him. "I just knew he wasn't going to be with us for a long time and I was just hoping I was wrong about it," she said. "I used to tell him stories about all these people that had died: my mother who had passed away, a cousin of mine who died when he was very young. I was almost fitting a lifetime in even in those early weeks. I'd tell him, 'You had a grandma who did this, and a cousin who did that, and I'm your mother who does this. . . .' It wasn't postpartum depression, this was a real fear. . . . Even when I was pregnant," Ellen recalled, "my best friend said that I never made plans for that baby. I never said, 'Gee, if it's a boy maybe he'll grow up to be a doctor, or if it's a girl, maybe she'll grow up to be President.' It wasn't an intentional thing. But my friend said that it always struck her as funny that I never made plans. I guess it was as though he was too good to be true. He was so perfect and so beautiful and so good, that it was almost as though this was too good to happen to us. That doesn't make a lot of sense, but that was the way I felt."

She had no reason for her feelings, but then feelings do not necessarily have a lot to do with reason. Both Ellen, a secretary in a congressman's office, and Jeff, a specialist in photographic processes for a federal agency in Washington, D.C., were healthy. And the five-pound, ten-ounce baby boy born August 28, 1979—five days shy of his parents' fifth anniversary—at first appeared to be healthy and normal in all respects. "He did all of the things little babies do," Ellen recalled. "He slept well, he ate well, there was some interest in some toys.

"Justin was four months old and he had rolled over a couple of times," Ellen said, "and then he stopped rolling over. We didn't think too much of it at the time except to remark to each other, 'Gee, he isn't doing that anymore, or he hasn't done that in a long time.' By the time he was about six months old and he wasn't sitting up and he wasn't rolling over—and I'm the oldest of seven children and I know a lot of things that babies do—I kept saying to the doctor, 'Justin's not doing this and he's not doing that and he's not getting up on his knees,' and every well-baby visit it was, 'Is he doing this?' and I would go, 'No, no, no, no, no,' and the pediatrician would say, 'Well, you know a lot of babies are late.'

"When Justin was ten months old Jeff went to his well-baby visit with me. The doctor was examining Justin and he said, 'He's got great muscle control and great torso control,' and Jeff looked up at him and he said, 'Well, then why doesn't he sit up?' At which point the doctor said, 'Maybe we should have him checked by a neurologist.' Up until that point I was a neurotic mother. As soon as Dad comes in it's 'Maybe something's wrong, we'd better have it checked,' " Ellen said, laughing, with a trace of bitterness in the laugh.

"Once we got into the testing, we were hoping for something that was curable," Jeff said.

"I was hoping for a brain tumor," said Ellen, only half joking. "At least I figured that was curable. We thought maybe it was muscular dystrophy and he'd need physical therapy. As we got into testing we weren't thinking about anything fatal. I felt I wasn't doing enough for him, I initially felt I wasn't giving him enough stimulation, which wasn't true."

On Thursday, July 3, 1980, Jeff and Ellen took Justin to Georgetown University Medical Center for an examination by a neurologist recommended by Justin's pediatrician. The neurologist "did a lot of typical tests to see what kind of motor skills he had, and muscle tone," Jeff said, "and then he looked in his eyes. Georgetown being a teaching hospital, he must have had five, six, seven people he called in to have them look in Justin's eyes. Here you have a ten-month-old baby who doesn't want anybody looking in his eyes, and he'd squirm around while they were holding him. Finally we took him away, we took him out of their arms and said, 'That's enough.' When it got to be like the fourth or fifth time, I pulled one of the students over and said, 'What are you looking at?' And she said something about the cornea and the rods and cones in his eye and made something up. But with my photography background I knew that what they said wasn't true, and what they told me was just something to put me off." (What Jeff didn't know at the time was that the neurologist had called the residents in to observe the cherry-red spot in the eye that is seen in Tay-Sachs children.)

"When we went back to his office, the neurologist essentially said, 'There's some problems, but there's no rush to confirm a diagnosis; bring him back whenever you feel like it for some tests,'" Jeff recalled. "At the time we didn't know that he knew then, but he would have let us come in a couple of weeks later—"

"A couple of months later," interjected Ellen. "That gave us a very false sense of security, because every time you're sent to a specialist with your child, an alarm goes off. You don't think he's going to die necessarily, but an alarm goes off...." The Fleishers went to Virginia Beach for the Fourth of July weekend, but had Justin back for testing on July 7. "I remember that that was the worst day of my life, the worst day," said Ellen, who explained that Justin was given a CAT scan, an EEG and other tests, even though, as she was to realize a short time later, Justin's problem had already been diagnosed.

On the morning of July 8, as Ellen stood beside the crib in Justin's hospital room, the neurologist entered the room and got right to the point. " 'Well, Mrs. Fleisher,' " she will always remember him saying, " 'it's one of three things.' I don't remember what the other two were but he said, 'Tay-Sachs,' and I looked at him and I said, 'You mean that my son is going to die?' And he said, 'I don't want to talk about that now. What time is your husband coming?' I said, 'Wait! You're telling me that my baby—the only thing I know about Tay-Sachs is that it's fatal.'

32

And he said, 'Well, what time is your husband coming?' And I said 'Eleven-thirty,' and he turned and walked out. Not a nurse came, not a doctor, not a priest, nobody! Nobody came, and we even had our own room. I mean I was all alone. His bedside manner was very poor. Even five years later I can say, 'Well, doctors are taught to heal and they don't know what to do with the dead and the dying,' but that's no excuse. When Jeff came in—I'd been hysterical all morning, running from Justin's room to the bathroom, screaming at God, saying all these horrible things. When Jeff came in, I looked at him and I said, 'All I know is that this child is going to die, he's going to die!' And I was right."

"None of the doctors ever did say he was going to die, [despite the fact that Tay-Sachs disease is always fatal, usually before age five]," said Jeff. "We'd say, 'He's going to die, isn't he?' And the neurologist would say, 'Well, everybody dies. The length of life is variable.' He said everything, but he never said he was going to die. He alluded to it, he said Justin was going to have a short-ened life, he said everything but."

"We were desperate for information," said Ellen, her frustra-tion still evident five years later. "There are some families that don't want to know. All they can absorb is that their child has a terminal illness. I was crazy trying to find out what was going to happen because I had no knowledge of the disease—and nobody would tell me anything.

"My friend called up the local chapter [of the Tay-Sachs Foundation] in Washington, and when she came to visit me that afternoon she said, 'Find out if Justin's going to go blind.' She knew the answer but she wanted me to ask the hospital. And I did that. I went up to the nurses' station, and this was the day of the diagnosis, and I said, 'Is Justin going to go blind?' and the nurse looked at me and she said, 'Of course he is.' That's how I found out that good piece of news.

33

"And the next morning the neurologist came in and asked if I would bring Justin in to show his residents. And being in a state of shock I said yes, I would do that. And I brought him in and he showed Justin's lack of development and turned him belly over and this child just flopped."

The following day Ellen and Jeff Fleisher left Georgetown with little information other than the fact that their first-born son was suffering from a fatal genetic disease. There had been no special counseling, no discussion with the doctor. "I think the head nurse expressed her sympathy," Ellen said. "Essentially we were sent home with him to die. We didn't have any information about the disease. I think we were still in shock when we got home. God, we ate out a lot! I became a nonperson. We were caught up in Justin and what was happening. I was like a Stepford wife, I just went through my routine. I made lunch at noon and I made dinner at five-thirty. We were concerned about how everyone else was taking the news. I had called my father (my mother had died when I was very young). We had enough presence of mind to say we had to keep going. Jeff had to go to work and I had to get up in the morning and get dressed. I had Jeff call my father to see how he was doing. But, you know, after a while you look at everybody else and you say, 'You have to handle this by yourself, our pain is horrible, we can't take your pain.' But originally it's 'How are you? We're okay. Are you okay?' "

Jeff added: "You get your strength from each other, you can't get it from somebody outside. Everybody tries to push you on social workers and counselors."

Ellen recalled that on the night of July 8, the day she had been told that Justin had Tay-Sachs, but the day before his discharge from the hospital, she had gone home for the night with Jeff and had left Justin alone. "I had a very good friend who said, 'That was horrible, you should have stayed with your son.' And I said, 'Justin is going to die and my husband is going to be left here, and we have a life we have to live together.' And even though Justin was responsive, very responsive, and knew who I was and knew I wasn't there that night, I had to be with my husband, and I think it was the first time that you cried," she said, turning toward Jeff. "That whole day you watched me and you supported me and I was an idiot. But that was the first time you had been able to break down, and I knew that if I had not gone home with him that night out lives would never be the same. . . . But I was just trying to cope, to accept it. . . . Not accept it, I don't know, I think that I was just getting into my routine, I was clinging to my order of life. I'd get up every morning with Justin and he had his breakfast and I had my breakfast and we went through our days, for maybe a month."

During that first month Ellen and Jeff returned to Georgetown for a final visit, for genetic counseling. It was then that they learned about Tay-Sachs, the genetic condition that affects and kills one of every 3600 children born to couples of Eastern European Jewish extraction. "I had heard of Tay-Sachs," Ellen recalled, "but I don't know how I heard of it. We had the confirmation of my pregnancy when I was four months pregnant. My obstetrician asked me if there was Tay-Sachs in the family and I said, 'No,' and he said, 'Well, then it's not necessary to be tested.' That is a very big complaint of parents in our groups, because very often there is no case of Tay-Sachs in the family. Today, if a patient even sounds as if they have a Jewish name they're told go get tested."

As part of their genetic counseling, the couple constructed a pedigree chart and "went back seventy-five years and found no Tay-Sachs on either side of the family," Ellen said.

But at that time, Jeff said, "We found that my mother had two brothers that died when they were very small children. We tracked down their death certificates: One died of leukemia and one died of scurvy. We thought it might be Tay-Sachs, because

35

Tay-Sachs victims don't eat. But the child died at nine months or so, so we really don't know. . . ."

"We couldn't go back very far into our families," Ellen continued, "because we have the same problem a lot of families do: Grandparents are alive and that's it, and their memories aren't very clear. My maiden name is Kravetz. We went back to our grandparents. Actually, my great-grandparents on my mother's side came from a town in Lithuania where some researchers thought they had isolated Tay-Sachs. There's some Holy Roller story about a sunspot that appeared and mutated all of these people's genes in this little town. We can't prove that medically, of course."

"My grandparents were the ones that came over to this country," Jeff said. "My father's parents came from Poland. My grandfather came over first, just before World War I. He served in World War I, and then he brought over my grandmother. His name was Morris Fleisher, and her name was Etta. They happened to be first cousins, but we don't think that's involved with the Tay-Sachs gene."

Knowing that their child was genetically sentenced to death changed Jeff and Ellen's attitude toward Justin. "For me it became more of a maintenance feeling," said Jeff. "He was still alive and everything, but there was no longer any kind of long-term plan. At that point you take care of him and everything and he's still pretty much a normal baby. As it went on, and it got worse and worse, you really have—what do you call it—you get negative feelings." He admitted that he occasionally thought about things like mercy killing. "All those thoughts go through your mind. I don't think it ever became a chore to care for Justin, I think what it is is that you gave him a bath and you know the suffering and everything and, I hate to say it, but you literally think, 'Well, I could turn this kid over and I could drown him,' and you really think you want to do that, but then you don't because you think, 'Well, it's not the right thing to do it.' At that time, when you're sitting there, you're very tempted to do something like that."

"I think you divorced yourself from him when he was diagnosed," Ellen told Jeff. "As you say, he died that day and you looked at him differently, your hopes and your dreams for him died that day. He said, 'I'm never going to go to Boy Scout camp with him and we're never going to go canoeing together and he's never going to see a sunrise.' "

"I was more concerned for him, my bad feelings were more he's never going to go to Scout camp, he's never going to go canoeing. That's what was really hard for me," Jeff responded. "That's sort of how I looked at it, it was over, at that point it was over, I knew he was going to die, and I was more upset not for myself that he was going to die but that he was going to miss these things." On reflection, however, Jeff is willing to acknowledge that the "pain" of Justin's deterioration was Jeff's, rather than Justin's. "I don't think he ever physically suffered," he said. "It was my pain, but that was at home. But when he was in the center in Virginia there were times when we walked in there, and although everybody always said he didn't feel any pain, his face was contorted, and he had tremors, and then I thought about [killing Justin], but it was for him."

"I never thought about putting a bag over Justin's head until he was at the center," Ellen began. She paused for a moment, and then corrected herself, saying, "That's really not true, because he would have crying jags at home. These children sometimes don't know when they're crying, they go over a line and they're inconsolable, and I would walk him and I would rock him and I would do everything and there was no way to comfort him for hours on end. I used to call up a friend of mine and say, 'I'm going to put a bag over the kid's head, I can't stand it anymore!' But that was my pain, my pain was, 'If you're going to die, die,'

37

and a lot of us who have children who are terminally ill say, well, 'If you're going to die, die, don't wait three years, or five years—if you're going to go, go, don't make it hard on everybody.' It's not that we didn't care. The pro-lifers are out there saying, 'You only care about your own pain,' which is very real, but we didn't want to see him be uncomfortable and die that way, it was a very undignified way, we felt that if he was going to die. . . .

"I think, as Jeff is talking about the maintenance of Justin, that Tay-Sachs children are very hard to feed, and there's two-hour feedings and three-hour feedings, and all-day bottles just to get an ounce into them, and I used to say, 'Why am I doing this? Why am I feeding this child? Why am I beating my head against a wall saying, You have to have a jar of baby food because you're ten months old, dammit! and that's what you're supposed to be eating.' "

Justin's Tay-Sachs was diagnosed in July, and by year's end his health had deteriorated markedly. "His vision was very poor and his feedings were taking us about two hours, he was severely constipated and I think he had just started having his seizures. He had three or four declines and then he would plateau. That's where it was a quick progression," Ellen said.

The difficulty in feeding Jusin marked the beginning of the end of his days at home. "The little bit of information we got from the hospital on the day of diagnosis indicated that he was going to need to be tube-fed," Ellen said, "and I said to Jeff, 'When Justin has to be tube-fed I don't want him at home anymore.' A lot of people make a lot of statements when their child is diagnosed, some will say, 'I'm never going to institutionalize him, I'm always going to keep him at home.' But I was very true to my word: that when he needed to be tube-fed, that was no longer emotionally—'satisfying' isn't the word I want—I could no longer handle that emotionally. And I always knew I was very traumatized by the fact that he was going to have to be tube-fed. He began to dehydrate when he was eighteen months old. We were getting food into him but no liquid, his sucking reflex was diminishing. I took him to the pediatrician and he said, 'Unless you can get liquid into him he's going to need the tube.' So by then we had had eight months of talking about it. We had very dear friends we had met through the Tay-Sachs group who lived in Virginia and who had placed their Tay-Sachs child in the same institution we were going to put Justin in. So we had had those eight months to see the facility, the Northern Virginia Training Center for the Retarded. They helped us get him in because there's so much red tape. Northern Virginia Training Center for the Retarded." So in February 1981, when Justin had to have a feeding tube surgically implanted, the Fleishers were ready to place their son in an institution.

Ellen said she did not want to give up Justin, but added: "I knew what my limits were. I didn't have any problem with those limits then, but when I think about it now, he was a very easy child to take care of: He did not have pneumonia; he did not have to be suctioned. He needed maintenance, he needed to be turned, he needed to be fed, and looking back I could have done it physically, but I still don't think I could have done it emotionally. I think that would have destroyed our lives."

"Physically you can do that," Jeff explained. "The mother sleeps in the room with the child and the father sleeps in their room. You can physically do all that, nurses can do it and you can do it. But what kind of quality of life is that, not only for the child, but for us, too?"

"I was his mother," Ellen said. "I just couldn't do that."

"I think our big thing was we knew in the back of our mind he would need twenty-four-hour care, and at the center the nurses are there twenty-four hours and we couldn't do that at home," Jeff added.

B. D. COLEN

Assuming that a couple is as lucky as Jeff and Ellen and can find a clean, caring, enlightened institution in which to place their disabled or dying child, they are almost immediately confronted by the staggering cost of such care. "I guess things were good and bad," said Jeff, explaining the arrangements that had to be made to pay for Justin's institutionalization. "At that time I had high-option Blue Cross/Blue Shield coverage under the federal plan, and they paid one hundred percent of all medical costs and hospitalization. But the one thing they don't pick up is when you actually place the child at the center. At that time the cost at the center was seventy-five dollars a day, which can really mount up. And it's on a sliding scale, depending upon your financial situation, and then you split the cost with Medicaid. I had to go to court to petition the court to get him into the center—essentially you're committing a child to an institution—and when you do that you become eligible for Medicaid and SSI [Social Security Supplemental Income] benefits." So Jeff, who earned about $30,000 a year, received $25 a month in SSI benefits for Justin's personal effects and ended up paying $140 a month toward the $2250 monthly bill for Justin's care. Medicaid paid the rest.

"It was not easy" to whittle the bill down that low, Jeff said. "If we'd had to pay the full seventy-five dollars a day we'd have been bankrupt very quickly. But in order to end up paying about five dollars a day. . . . We were very lucky. I forget who told us this, but the state looks at all your assets and your debts at that time, and that's how they decide what you're going to pay. So we essentially had to get rid of all our money, all our assets—you're either going to have to pay it to the state or you pay it to something else. He [Justin] was going to get the same care no matter what, so we went out and bought furniture and bought a bunch of stuff to use up our free cash, essentially. We had to quick get some debts. My feeling was I'd rather use that money to buy

40

some furniture than give it to the state. We bought a new car, because I'd totaled the car about three weeks before he was admitted. Maybe it was a bad attitude to have, but. . . ."

Ellen said that even though she knew she couldn't care for Justin at home, and even though the infirmary room in which he lived was a cheerful, bright place with yellow walls and children's decorations, placing him there was "very difficult."

"I had no other children and I went home to an empty crib, and that was devastating to me that the room was bare, there was no child in there," she said. "I used to think I heard him in the middle of the night and I would say to Jeff, 'Justin's crying, you have to go get him,' because he would get up in the morning he wouldn't remember that he had gotten up in the middle of the night, where as if I got up at two A.M. I was up at two A.M. . . . Or I would go running in in the middle of the night after Justin had been placed and I would stand in the doorway realizing that he wasn't home. And that was a very hard thing for me to do, to deal with that. It took me a long time before I could go in there and clean up his room, and empty out his drawers, and leave the door open . . . it was months."

But Ellen would visit Justin every day at the center. "He could hear, but he couldn't see. He was blind by then. He knew who I was. I'd go at lunchtime and stay a couple of hours. Some days they could get him to suck on his bottle. They made the hole in the nipple much larger. His sucking reflex was totally diminished, but I could hold him and rock him and give him the bottle. Even though I accepted it, I know this is contradictory, but I couldn't believe this was happening to him, that he was there, that I was doing it. It became a routine to me. I'd get up every morning, I'd get dressed, I'd do the dishes, and I'd go. It was my life. And I used to get into bed at night and I'd never thought we would be able to live one day at a time like they tell you, and it's a horrible saying and everybody hates it that goes through this, but you'd get to bed at the end of the day and say, 'Thank you for letting me get through the day.' It's so draining."

Jeff visited his son about once a week, on Sunday afternoons. "I'd hold him in the rocking chair and watch a football game or something," he said. "You're sort of in a daze—you're holding him, and you look at him, but you almost had like this little brick wall that you built up: He's your son, but he isn't your son, it's hard to describe. . . ."

"We'd lost him," Ellen said. "He wasn't the way we thought things were going to be with him."

"Because of the place where he was, a mental institution," Jeff continued, "a lot of times you'd see these other kids in the infirmary, because they were sick or something, and you'd see them strapped into their chairs and you'd look at Justin and you were almost sort of happy he was going to die; we were almost thankful for us that it was going to end."

Ellen added: "I was very thankful he was not going to end up a drooling nineteen-year-old person that had to be strapped in a chair to sit up and had to have someone to feed him. I was glad he was not going to have to live like that."

At the time Justin was placed, Ellen was trying to get pregnant again. "We had decided after Justin was initially diagnosed that we wanted a family. I was, and I still am, very angry at God, and I thought, 'You're not going to beat me on this—I'm going to have my family whether you like it or not. If I have to have fifty-two abortions I'm going to have my family.' We wanted a family, it was very important to us. So we took the advice of a very good friend who said, 'Go home and have another baby, not as a replacement for Justin, but if you wait till he dies, God forbid but he could be seven—what are you waiting for?' For us that was very good advice—a lot of parents don't like that advice, but we needed that, we needed to hear from somebody that 'I have three healthy children, or two healthy children,' and that's what we did."

This time the Fleishers knew to go through prenatal screening and were ready to face an abortion if necessary. "I always felt abortion was not right for contraception," Ellen said. "My idea was that if you got pregnant by accident, once maybe was okay, but let's not make a practice of this. But I really was not involved with it, I never really gave it much thought. But after Justin was diagnosed, there was no doubt I would never, ever go through that again, and I would never have a child that would go through that again. We talked a lot about aborting, a lot. We never talked about things like 'What are we going to name the baby?'—you can't when you find out in a situation like that. We talked a lot about abortion. We talked about what the abortion was going to be like (because I was going to have to have a C-section)."

"You don't think about the baby, you don't really enjoy a pregnancy until you know," Jeff said. "You don't think about names, you don't make any plans, you don't decorate the room. For Justin, we had the room and everything decorated like a month after we found out we were pregnant. With this pregnancy, we didn't do anything until we found out. We used Justin's room for Brent because Justin had the second biggest room and we redecorated it a little bit to make it different for him. But we didn't do a thing until we got those results."

Ellen had her amniocentesis at Johns Hopkins Hospital in Baltimore, rather than at Georgetown, which had such bad memories associated with it, and both Ellen and Jeff were at home when the call came with the test results. "I ran out front and yelled, 'The baby's okay!' I was an idiot," Ellen recalled. "For that pregnancy we had told a lot of our friends and a lot of our neighbors because we needed that support, that help to get through. Those were tears of joy. We were just elated. I called up my father and he answered the phone and I said to him, 'The baby's okay,' and he stopped a minute because I think he thought that Justin was okay. And there was a very long pause,

43

and a great hesitation from him, until he realized I didn't mean that my baby Justin was okay, I meant that the baby I was carrying was okay . . . [then] he was delighted."

Brent Fleisher, a normal, healthy boy, was born August 31, 1981, three days after Justin's second birthday. Justin was still responsive at that point, but because of a complication related to her cesarean, Ellen was unable to visit him for about three weeks after Brent's birth. "When I went back to see him I felt that he didn't know who I was anymore. That spark, where I could walk into his room and he would smile—whether it was my voice or my perfume, I don't know what—was gone." At that point Ellen stopped her daily visits, and instead would go to the center every couple of days with Justin's new brother. "Brent would sit in the infant seat and I would hold Justin," she said. "Sometimes I would put Brent at the end of the bed in Justin's crib and take Justin out of the crib and hold him."

Ellen said the birth of Brent did nothing to change her feelings toward Justin, but it did soften the blow of his impending death. "Dealing with Justin was easier. Brent softened the blow a little bit. We've always said Brent and then Adam [the Fleishers' third son] were our commitments to survival. They really gave us, not meaning, that sounds very dramatic, but reason to go on. It's devastating to lose a child, and they gave us something to cling to, a life to cling to. I remember saying to Jeff that when Brent was born finally the house would scream with tears of joy and laughter, rather than sadness."

"It was a lot more fun to go to the center, if you can call it fun," Jeff added. "We'd put Brent in the crib and he'd crawl around and pull Justin's hair, pull the tube." Ellen and Jeff both laughed. "It's awful to laugh about," she said, "but it broke the tension."

Within four months of Brent's birth Ellen was again pregnant. "We did it that quick because we didn't know if it would be

Tay-Sachs again and we'd have to abort. We didn't want to stretch it out too far," Jeff said. But son Adam, who was born September 16, 1982, was also normal, which helped the couple to deal with the horror of Justin's final months.

"I remember we were sort of racing the clock," Jeff continued. "I'd always wanted a picture of the three boys together so that the other two would have that." So when Adam was about three weeks old, the parents took Brent and Adam to the center for a visit. Justin was drifting in and out of coma by that time. His coloring was blue, he was constantly drooling, and he had to have artificial tears placed in his eyes because he was no longer blinking. "When we first placed him we had a session with the doctors discussing extraordinary measures," Jeff said. "We decided not to do any extraordinary measures and we had to write them a letter saying that we give our permission that no extraordinary measures be used in case he stops breathing or something like that. But the doctor always said he reserved the right to administer medication and things like that and he said he always reserved the last word but he would take our wishes into account. I always objected to that because I said as father, I should have the last word. But we never clashed on that. . . ." For in his three years of dying, Justin never had pneumonia, never needed antibiotics and only needed an occasional baby aspirin for the fever associated with minor infections.

"He was the most healthy dying child you've ever seen," joked Ellen, who said that, toward the end, she was only visiting Justin once a week. "I called every day, but it was getting very hard to go. If he wasn't my son, I don't know if I'd have visited him."

"We wouldn't stay very long," Jeff said. "At that time you couldn't pick him up or anything, either. He was very sensitive. If you touched his leg it would stiffen up and there'd be a tremor."

"It wasn't worth it," Ellen interjected.

"We'd see him," Jeff continued, "make sure he was all right, change the diaper under his head because it was always wet. . . ."

On Monday, January 10, 1983, the physician at the center called the Fleisher home, which was about forty minutes from the institution. "Justin had taken kind of a turn, and it's probably another week or two," Ellen said they were told. "It's very hard. You always want a doctor to say the day your child is going to die is this date at this time, and of course nobody can do that. And we had never gotten a call in the two years he was there. He said it's probably a week, maybe two, there's no need to come now. But that night Jeff and I went. Tuesday morning the doctor called me and he said, 'I have never seen a child deteriorate as rapidly as Justin has.' He was vomiting blood."

"When we went there Tuesday morning, that's when we saw he was very blue, he was tired. The change from Monday night was amazing," said Jeff.

Said Ellen: "We looked at death."

The couple stayed by Justin's bedside all day, leaving about 6 P.M. to get some dinner. "I knew this was it," said Jeff. He turned toward Ellen: "When he was first born you knew he wasn't going to have a long life. That day I knew that was it." Ellen and Jeff had dinner at a nearby restaurant and then went home briefly to check on Brent and Adam. Then they returned to the center.

"It was very important for us to be with Justin when he died," his mother said. "Jeff experienced the loss of grandparents, but he never experienced the loss of an immediate family member. He, more so than I was, was very afraid of death, so it was very important for us to be there. And thankfully, Justin had a very peaceful death. But we were always worried he was going to choke to death, he was going to choke on his vomit. We had this horrible vision of him gasping for air, of him clutching at the air, and thankfully we did not see what we had imagined was going to happen."

"I got up and walked out, and about ten seconds after I did the nurse came out and said he's not breathing," Jeff recalled. "I came back into the room and I saw him actually die."

"Maybe I walked in at that point," Ellen said. "I walked over to the crib and I kissed him, and I said to you, he let out this very deep sigh."

"Everybody was just sort of standing there," Jeff continued the story. "Then this nurse said, 'I guess I'd better listen for a heartbeat.' Then they had to call a doctor." Justin's body was bathed and dressed in pajamas his parents had long before chosen for his burial.

Despite saying that she was "relieved" when Justin died, Ellen said: "When they came from the funeral home and they were ready to take him, I looked at the man and said, 'Give me another minute.' I said, 'I want one more minute.' It's ironic that all of this time we knew he was going to die, and I didn't have enough time. Then I walked into the room and said, 'This is stupid,' but we couldn't be there when they took him away. But the worst thing, though, that day, was walking back into the room after they had taken Justin and the crib had already been stripped, with new sheets on it. It was very disturbing to me that five minutes before my son had lay dead there, and then it was as though he was gone. That was very disturbing to me."

Jeff and Ellen were almost through mourning for Justin by the time he died, for their mourning had begun that July day so long ago when the neurologist had first spoken the words "Tay-Sachs." "We grieved from the time he was diagnosed until the time he died," the mother said, "and I think, by the time he died we looked at each other and we said, 'How many more tears? How many more tears can you shed?' It was enough after two and one-half years." The earlier mourning, she explained, was "not the mourning that you would have when somebody dies and you go to the funeral. I think you do mourn at that point, you mourn for those couple of years when he's still alive. I think we felt worse then than when he really died. I think we were all 'mourned out' then, if you will. I think you do go through a mourning; well, we always say that these children die three times: They die when they're diagnosed, they die when they're placed in an institution—if you do that—and they die when they really die. After the diagnosis you don't think of it as mourning, but you're so depressed, you go through all those feelings, that by the time he really dies you don't have that anymore to go through. You really do mourn during that middle phase."

"We had the funeral and all the relatives came down and—it was like just another day for us really, it was literally like another day," Jeff said. "Everybody else was all upset, and we had a hard time understanding why they were so upset. We were more relieved than anything else."

Said Ellen: "It was over for him and over for us."

"He looked more peaceful right after he died than he had done for a long time, so it was a very positive and very good feeling, not a negative feeling," Jeff added.

"Soon after the diagnosis, like a week or two, Jeff went to camp with my father and I had gone to Rochester with Justin," Ellen recalled, "and I was crying and I was grieving and my stepmother said to me, 'How can you be grieving for him, he's still here. You should wait until after he dies.' And it's very hard for anyone else to understand that there was that horrible grief, and even though he was alive, we were grieving for him. It's silly when people say, 'Go home and enjoy what you can,' and yet I will say to new parents, 'Take a lot of pictures and enjoy what you can get out of these children now, because when they're not responsive anymore, and they don't smile at you anymore, and they don't know who you are anymore, it's horrible, it's a horror. Try to appreciate what they are doing, and what your relationship is with them and cling to that, but it's hard to have good times after that with the children."

In April 1984, Ellen Fleisher became pregnant for the fourth time. By then, a new prenatal diagnostic test, chorionic villus sampling, was just becoming available, a procedure that could be undertaken in the tenth week of pregnancy, rather than the sixteenth to eighteenth like amniocentesis and one that can produce genetic information about the fetus almost immediately. "The biggest consideration in our getting pregnant again was the availability of this test," Ellen said. "I had heard too many stories of parents having abortions at six months and delivering stillborns." So Jeff and Ellen went to Philadelphia to one of the few facilities then testing the procedure. By the time they arrived back in Washington, about 6 P.M. the same evening, Dr. Laird Jackson, who had done the testing, was calling with the results.

As Jeff remembered that phone call, Jackson "was sort of stumbling over his words, but he said it was a Tay-Sachs fetus. He was very gentle and kind about it, but very matter-of-fact."

"I think that after Jeff got off the phone with Dr. Jackson my initial reaction was that, again, we'd lost control," Ellen said. "Everybody wants to have control of their lives, and we'd lost such a great amount of control with Justin. And Jeff kept saying, 'You don't have a choice, there is nothing to discuss, you have to abort this fetus, we've already decided that.' And I said, 'But I want a choice,' I still wanted somebody to say to me, 'Do you want to have this done?' But there was no choice. We knew we didn't want to have another Justin, we knew we didn't want to have another child go through that ever again. But I felt, again somebody has made this choice for me. But we had always said Justin began to die the moment he was conceived, and this little fetus had begun to die the moment he was conceived. It was hard for us. We knew it was a life. But it was a death also. We never found out about the sex of that last pregnancy.

"Religiously, we consider ourselves traditionalists," Ellen said.

"We're what my grandfather would call 'holiday Jews'—he was a rabbi in Rochester—but Jeff likes to say that when God comes down and apologizes for taking Justin, he'll consider religion. I don't believe the way I used to believe, which is why when Brent asked me, 'Mommy, what is God?' I couldn't answer the way my mother used to answer me that God is all-loving and all-caring and he takes care of us all and he loves all the children and he protects us. I don't think God is so terrific, that he makes the sick babies better and you only die when you're old.

"In fact," Ellen Fleisher summed up, "I will always be angry at God. Sometimes I think God will be very afraid to meet me because I have quite a few things to say."

CHAPTER 2

Engineering Health

Imagine, for a moment, an enormous, complex, jigsaw puzzle, dumped out of its box onto a large tabletop. In the far left-hand corner of the table is a mountain of pieces, not yet identified, in all shapes, colors and sizes. Around the edges of the table are forty-six smaller piles of pieces that the person working the puzzle has identified as somehow belonging together. Within this perimeter of piles are a few very short stretches of border worked out, but those tiny straight lines serve only to stress the complexity of the task that lies ahead. And within the sketchy outline of the broken border are a handful of little sections that have been pieced together, but most of these sections lie far from each other on the empty ocean of the tabletop.

There is such a puzzle, and it lies in similarly chaotic disarray on laboratory benches at institutions such as MIT, Cold Spring Harbor Laboratory, the National Cancer Institute, the University of California at San Francisco, Harvard, Columbia and the Wistar Institute. At these and dozens of other centers of molecular and developmental biology, researchers are attempting to piece together this puzzle that is the human genome, the billions of molecules of deoxyribonucleic acid that make up the genes that make up the chromosomes that make us all at once astoundingly similar and dissimilar.

The forty-six small sections of the puzzle that have been pieced together are the chromosomes, together carrying all the genetic information necessary for the production of a human being. The chromosomes are largely made up of segments of DNA molecules, called genes, and each of these segments in turn carries the code for a particular protein needed to produce a human cell or to keep that cell functioning properly. The researchers working on the puzzle today know the shapes of these forty-six pieces. They can even see them under a microscope. They know that certain of the puzzle's basic pieces, the genes, belong on certain chromosomes. Additionally, they understand some of the functions associated with each chromosome and some of the functions associated with the individual genes. But that is a far cry from knowing what the entire puzzle looks like or how the entire genome functions.

In fact, what is remarkable today is not how much is known about human genetics, but how little is known in this scientific era in which man has eliminated smallpox from the face of the earth and can design and program computers to perform computational tasks hitherto beyond human reach. This does not mean that great strides have not been made, for they have. It was only about one hundred and twenty years ago, after all, that Gregor Mendel, an Austrian monk with a fondness for gardening, first took the puzzle off the shelf and provided the theory of how it might go together. And literally every day, in a laboratory somewhere in the scientific world, another minute piece of the puzzle is at least identified, if not completely understood. But the puzzle is so complex, so mind-bogglingly enormous, that it will be at least decades before it is completed—if it is ever completed.

Tay-Sachs disease, which claimed the life of Justin Fleisher and that of one in every 3600 children of couples of Ashkenazi

Jewish extraction, is one of a number of so-called single-gene disorders: those caused by a single defective gene. Tay-Sachs disease is a perfect example of a single-gene disorder and of the kind of havoc caused by the absence or less than optimal functioning of just one of the approximately 50,000 genes in each human cell. Tay-Sachs is what is called an autosomal recessive genetic disorder. That is, for a child to develop Tay-Sachs, *both* parents must be carriers of the Tay-Sachs trait. In a normal individual there are two genes, one from each parent, whose function is to produce the enzyme hexosaminidase A (hex-A), the absence of which causes Tay-Sachs. A Tay-Sachs carrier has one gene that produces hex-A normally and one Tay-Sachs gene, and the one properly functioning gene is enough for normal function. But each time two carriers have a child, there is a one-in-four chance the child will have Tay-Sachs, a one-in-four chance the child will be Tay-Sachs-free and a two-in-four chance the child will be a carrier. If the child is a carrier, its health will not be affected by Tay-Sachs, although it has a two-in-four chance of passing the Tay-Sachs gene on to *its* children.

But if the child has two Tay-Sachs genes, it will suffer the awful fate of Justin Fleisher. For the role of the Tay-Sachs gene in the genetic scheme of things is to produce hex-A, which clears a fatty substance called ganglioside GM_2 from cells, especially those of the central nervous system. Without the action of hex-A, this fatty buildup in the brain cells begins during fetal development and continues until the child dies, invariably by about age five. Life begins normally for such children, but like Justin Fleisher, their neurological and motor development usually peak well before the first birthday. Rather than accomplishing more and more, as normal children do, the Tay-Sachs children appear able to do less and less. Complex motor functions, such as crawling, begin to disappear. Vision and hearing are impaired. Most such children are suffering seizures by the age of one.

53

To make the situation even more difficult, the most logical treatment, artificially producing hex-A and treating the children with it, has thus far proved impossible. The main problem has not been producing the enzyme. Rather, researchers have been stymied by the brain's ability to protect itself by means of something called the blood-brain barrier, which keeps foreign substances from reaching the brain cells. To treat Tay-Sachs victims successfully with the replacement enzyme, scientists must first develop a way to get that enzyme, or the gene to produce that enzyme, past the blood-brain barrier. And so today, abortion of affected fetuses is the only "treatment" for Tay-Sachs disease.

Between 2000 and 3000 single-gene conditions have been identified. Some of these diseases, such as sickle-cell anemia and cystic fibrosis, devastate the lives of thousands, if not millions, of individuals worldwide and are well known to the public. Others, such as adenosine deaminase deficiency (ADA), are only known to have affected fewer than 100 persons worldwide. Most of these conditions, in fact, are extremely rare, yet 1 to 2 percent of all infants are born suffering from one or another of these disorders caused by the absence or malfunctioning of a single tiny strand of DNA. Geneticists are now able to provide prenatal screening for about 10 percent of these conditions, as well as for a number of chromosomal abnormalities. Chromosomal defects, such as Down's syndrome, are caused by an absence of a piece of chromosome or the presence of an extra piece. These abnormalities occur in about one in 200 births and are thought to be responsible for as many as half of all miscarriages.

As recently as a single childbearing generation ago, pregnant women had little more information about the genetic health of the fetus they were carrying than their great-grandmothers had during *their* pregnancies. While there was little awareness among parents then of their particular risks of producing an infant with one of the thousands of genetic diseases, even if a couple knew that they carried the gene for sickle-cell anemia or Huntington's disease, there was nothing that could be done to screen their pregnancy to assure them that their child would not also be affected. Thus, the only thing a hemophiliac could do to make sure that he would not father a hemophiliac son was not to father any children. The only thing an Ashkenazi Jewish couple could do to be absolutely sure that they would not have a child with Tay-Sachs was to have no children. And then came amniocentesis and ultrasound.

With the introduction of amniocentesis in the late 1960s, and then ultrasonography a short time later, it became possible to, in effect, examine the developing fetus in utero for certain genetic defects. During the procedure known as amniocentesis, performed sometime between the sixteenth and eighteenth week of pregnancy, a long needle is inserted through the pregnant woman's abdomen, through her uterus and into the amniotic sac, and a small amount of amniotic fluid is withdrawn. This fluid contains cells shed by the fetus, and these cells are collected and then grown in a culture medium until there are enough to allow a geneticist to study the fetal chromosomes for defects. It is possible to identify a Tay-Sachs-affected fetus by the absence of hex-A in the cells. Additionally, it is possible through the use of genetic probes to screen the fetal DNA for specific single-gene defects. Ultrasonography involves a technology very similar to that used in sonar on submarines. A sound-emitting probe is passed back and forth over the pregnant woman's abdomen and the sound waves produce a "picture" of the fetus. While to the uninitiated these images may look like nothing so much as an extremely "snowy" television picture, ultrasonography has now been refined to the point where it can be used not only to count and examine fetal limbs and the gross fetal anatomy, but also to examine the functioning of the fetal heart valves and other internal structures.

But what good does all this screening do the pregnant mother? Unfortunately, as this is being written a woman who discovers she is carrying a fetus with a genetic defect is still in much the same position as the person putting together a massive jigsaw puzzle with a missing or damaged piece: She can complete the puzzle without the piece, and it will never look quite right; or she can throw out the puzzle because it has been ruined by the absence of the piece. Thus, the mother who is informed her fetus will suffer from Tay-Sachs disease, or Down's syndrome, or polycystic kidney disease, or Duchenne's muscular dystrophy is faced with a Hobson's choice: She can carry the fetus to term, knowing that, in the case of Tay-Sachs, her child will in all likelihood die before its fifth birthday, or she can have it aborted—and thus killed before it is born.

While such parents are certainly provided with a choice, medical science can offer them little beyond that choice. In most cases, death is the only available therapy. Imagine the public outcry if a prominent physician were to propose killing adults suffering from incurable physically or mentally debilitating conditions or those suffering from terminal illnesses. Just look at the outrage when Colorado Governor Richard Lamm did nothing other than sensibly suggest that the elderly should not seek to extend their dying process through heroic medical intervention but rather should make way for the living.

Standard therapies are available for some of those affected with the genetically linked disorders: Diabetics can be kept alive with insulin injections; hemophiliacs can survive with the help of clotting factors; the ravages of PKU (phenylketonuria) can be fended off with strict dietary controls. But all of these, and most other treatments, are half-measures. Diabetics, for instance, develop any number of complications, including possible blindness and eventual loss of limbs. Hemophiliacs are susceptible to any number of infections, including AIDS, carried by their donated clotting factor. And it's often difficult, if not impossible, to keep a small child on a strict PKU diet. Unfortunately, however, these half-measures are the best physicians can offer patients with these genetic diseases.

By the time you read these words, we may have entered yet another era of medical care, the age of gene therapy. For it is expected that certainly within the next five years, and perhaps as early as 1986, a physician-researcher will attempt, in a fully sanctioned experiment, to cure a genetic disease in a human patient by augmenting or replacing that patient's defective gene. The fact that such an experiment will be technically feasible immediately raises the question of whether it is an ethically or morally *right* thing to do. "Technology is not the source of ethics," notes Dr. John Fletcher, assistant for bioethics at the National Institutes of Health, "but it creates alternatives that you never had before, and you have to choose whether to act on one or more of these alternatives."

We are now at the point where some alternatives are being offered to us as realistic possibilities in the very near future. The choices we make in this area may have a profound impact on the very future of the human race as we know it, in terms both of what these decisions physically bring about and of the moral and ethical climate they create. But in order to make informed decisions, we must have at least a clear basic understanding of what it is we as a society are being asked to decide.

What, then, do we and don't we mean when we speak of "gene therapy"? There are two basic forms of gene therapy currently under discussion, somatic cell therapy and germ cell therapy, and both their end results and ethical implications are enormously different. Somatic cell therapy amounts to using a bit of genetic material to cure an individual patient of a disease. Germ cell therapy, on the other hand, would in theory permanently eliminate the genetic disease being treated from the patient's genetic complement. That is, the patient's genetic makeup would be altered in such a way by germ cell therapy that he or she would be cured of the condition and would not pass the defect on to future generations. Thus, it can be argued that, except for the fact that DNA is the "medicine," somatic cell therapy is little different from standard medical treatments in which a drug is used to cure a patient of a particular disease. Germ cell therapy, however, involves what some would call "playing God," altering the basic genetic makeup of a particular family and therefore of all humankind.

The basic mechanics of somatic cell gene therapy have been worked out for some time. The defective gene that causes a particular disease is identified and its normal equivalent is isolated and cloned, or copied. The properly functioning gene is then inserted into normal human cells in one of several ways: It can, quite literally, be injected; it can be inserted into a specially inactivated virus, which is then taken up by the cells; it can be placed in its own membrane, which is then attached to cells in the body, allowing the DNA to enter the body's cells; or it can be chemically treated to enter particular cells in the body. At this point, the two most promising techniques are the use of viruses as delivery vehicles and so-called microinjection. Of the two, viral insertion seems a more likely way to go, if for no other reason than that microinjecting DNA into each of several hundred, or thousand, individual cells is such a tedious process and ends up delivering far less "good" DNA to the target cells in the body than would viruses. Once the replacement gene is established in the body, it is supposed to reproduce itself, and whatever protein it produces is supposed to provide the regulation needed to cure or prevent the occurrence of the genetic disease caused by an absence of the protein. All of this, of course, depends upon the researcher's ability to get the right gene in the right place, have it reproduce, be able to turn it "on," and be able to turn it back off if necessary—no small order.

The concept of somatic cell gene therapy is more than just theory, however. Researchers have already successfully carried out somatic cell experiments by inserting human genes into animal cells. As early as 1982, Dr. Dusty Miller, of the Salk Institute in La Jolla, California, cloned the human gene that carries the code for the enzyme hypoxanthine-guanine phosphoribosyltransferase (HPRT). A lack of this enzyme is responsible for Lesch-Nyham syndrome, a condition generally known only to the parents of its young victims and those in the medical profession. There are no telethons for the estimated 200 Lesch-Nyham sufferers born every year. There are no poster children for a condition that causes mental retardation, cerebral palsy and horrendous self-mutilation—its child victims often attempt to bite off their own fingers.

The traditional approach to treating an enzyme deficiency such as Lesch-Nyham would be to attempt to artificially reproduce the enzyme whose deficiency causes the condition and then provide the victims with the enzyme. The treatment of diabetics, a disease that is genetically linked, though it is not caused by an enzyme deficiency, is an example of this concept at work: Diabetes is held in check by the artificial introduction into the body of the product the body fails to produce—insulin.

But here's where the dollar signs enter the equation. With a condition like diabetes, which has millions of victims, there are huge profits to be reaped by drug companies that produce insulin. But the wheels of the pharmaceutical industry are not driven by either altruism or a thirst for knowledge for knowledge's sake. The bottom line on a corporate balance sheet, not the image of a few hundred retarded children mutilating themselves, is what sets research priorities. Thus, the research director of a pharmaceutical firm would immediately dismiss from his mind any thought of devoting resources to an attempt to produce the enzyme to treat Lesch-Nyham syndrome, which affects only about 200 of the 3.5 million babies born each year in the United

States, or the enzyme needed by the 40 to 50 cases of adenosine deaminase deficiency (ADA) reported worldwide. So the only possible treatment for these children is gene therapy perfected by academic, rather than commercial, research scientists.

It looked for a while as though the first attempt at gene therapy would be made on a Lesch-Nyham patient, with researchers inserting cloned HPRT genes into stem cells in the bone marrow, where, theoretically, they would reproduce and eventually replace the malfunctioning genes. Undoubtedly, such an experiment will be attempted within the next few years, but it looks now as if one of the tiny handful of ADA patients will be the first to benefit from the authorized clinical trial of a gene therapy on a human.

Actually, this will not be the first attempt to correct a genetic defect in a human. In 1981, Dr. Martin Cline, a researcher at the University of California at Los Angeles medical school, made an *unauthorized* attempt to cure beta-thalassemia in two women, one in Israel and one in Italy. Beta-thalassemia is a single-gene disease that affects an estimated 100,000 persons born each year worldwide. Its victims, who are largely of Mediterranean descent, suffer from an inability of the blood to carry a sufficient amount of hemoglobin, and thus may suffer from severe anemia. Cline had applied for approval to two UCLA review panels, one overseeing human experimentation and one overseeing recombinant DNA experiments. And because he had federal funds, Cline also needed the approval of a National Institutes of Health oversight group. But the NIH group would not act without the prior approval of the local review boards, and the two UCLA review groups each refused to act until their NIH counterpart had granted approval. So rather than continue to fight his way through the bureaucracy, Cline sought and gained the approval of a hospital in Italy and a hospital in Israel and carried out his experiment abroad. He injected a cloned beta-globin gene into the bone marrow of each of his two patients, but the expected improvement failed to materialize. Rather than trigger an avalanche of similar experiments by other researchers, as did Christiaan Barnard's unsuccessful first human heart transplant, Cline's effort resulted instead in his losing about a half-million dollars in federal grants, his resigning from his UCLA administrative position and his being remembered as the researcher who failed before he should have tried.

If there is one lesson to be learned from the Cline debacle it is that—at least on this frontier of medical research, treatment and technology—there are myriad guidelines, federal agencies and advisory boards, and public and private watchdogs, all of them examining the ongoing research at each stage of development. The National Institutes of Health has a Recombinant DNA Advisory Committee, which in turn has a Working Group on Human Gene Therapy—any researcher who receives any federal funds must submit research proposals to this body for approval. Additionally, hospitals and universities all have their own federal review processes, including institutional review boards (IRBs), which must give prior approval to *all* research involving human subjects. Scientists working with recombinant DNA, and not just those who are working toward attempting human gene therapy, have been cognizant of the public's skittishness about genetic engineering. It was, after all, the scientists themselves who, in 1974, proposed a moratorium on research in recombinant DNA until it became clear that the work currently under way, and that proposed for the immediate future, appeared to pose little danger to society.

There are two principal reasons why the current efforts in human gene therapy should be viewed as little more dangerous than current medical therapy. First, the NIH guidelines for genetic therapy on humans require information about risk-assessment studies, public health considerations, informed consent, provision of accurate information to the public, "timely communication of research methods and results to investigators and clinicians" and the submission of the minutes of all local review boards that have considered the proposal. All of that is required in addition to the scientific detail one would assume would be reviewed prior to NIH approval. Second, and even more important, is the fact that at this point, no responsible researcher is seriously proposing human germ cell therapy. All current efforts are devoted to curing a single disease in a single individual, and it looks as if that is where all efforts will be directed for some time to come, for human germ cell therapy is not scientifically feasible at this time.

But that does not mean we can dismiss germ cell therapy from our minds and blithely assume that no one will ever attempt it. Whether or not human germ cell therapy ever becomes feasible and is attempted will in large part depend upon societal attitudes toward such work. And if there is any aspect of genetic engineering that raises questions about eugenics, the "betterment" of the species through the elimination of genetic "defects," it is germ cell therapy.

Germ cell therapy involves the alteration of the genetic complement in male sperm, in the female ova, or in the male or female cells that produce the sperm or ova. The process is complicated. Because millions of sperm are involved in each fertilization attempt, yet only one penetrates the egg, it would be necessary to replace the defective gene in *all* sperm being used in each fertilization. Obviously, it would therefore make more sense to isolate the single egg prior to conception, as is now done during the in vitro fertilization process, remove the nucleus of the egg and replace the defective gene. The egg could then be fertilized in vitro—in a glass dish—or it could be returned to the uterus or fallopian tube to be fertilized in the normal manner. The third possibility is to perform the genetic manipulation on the embryo in the first few hours or days of its development. This methodology is in itself controversial because it raises all the questions about the rights of the embryo and the ethics of experimenting with human embryos. Additionally, any method of germ cell therapy confronts the researcher or clinician with the problem of determining whether his gene replacement has "taken." Obviously, if a genetic defect is considered serious enough to attempt germ cell therapy in the first place, it is too serious to simply attempt the genetic repair and then allow the pregnancy to go to term without determining if the repair has been effective. Thus, germ cell therapy requires the same kind of fetal intervention, such as amniocentesis, as current prenatal screening and raises the same specter of abortion.

Then what is the "advantage," if any, of germ cell therapy? It would eliminate a genetic defect, such as Huntington's disease or Tay-Sachs, from a patient's entire germ line. Not only would the treated germ cells, or embryo, not develop into an infant with the disease, but the person who grew from those treated cells would not carry the defective gene and thus would not pass the defect on to future generations. So it is conceivably possible by using germ cell therapy to virtually eliminate single-gene defects in much the same way small pox was eradicated. However, universal screening is impossible, and it is equally impossible to prevent spontaneously arising defects. Thus, the disease could never be completely eliminated.

Would germ cell therapy work? The answer is a qualified yes. If the experiments of Richard D. Palmiter and Ralph L. Brinster are any indication, then germ cell therapy *might* someday work on humans. Palmiter and Brinster have on several occasions succeeded in altering the genetic makeup of mouse embryos and have traced those alterations through several succeeding generations. In one experiment they succeeded 6 percent of the time in injecting a rat growth hormone gene into mouse embryos. About one-third of the treated mice produced the growth hormone and developed into "super mice," twice the size of their untreated, or unsuccessfully treated, litter mates.

But the very success of the Palmiter-Brinster experiment raises the worst fears about human gene therapy. Do we want to produce the human equivalent of "super mice"? While the question may seem farfetched, is it farfetched to ask if we would want the human race free from most of the single-gene defects we know today? Dr. W. French Anderson, chief of the laboratory of molecular hematology at the National Heart, Lung and Blood Institute, thinks we do. "Ask every parent who has a defective child," replied Anderson, who is a member of the NIH's Working Group on Human Gene Therapy. "People who don't suffer always stand out and say this [germ cell therapy] is wrong. Yes, maybe a hundred generations from now we will be sorry" because we discover something good was eliminated from the germ line along with the defect, "but I don't know of a single physician in the world who does not want to eliminate genetic defects."

Not everyone is as sanguine about the idea as Anderson. "I feel that under the appropriate conditions, when it is safe for the individual, somatic cell therapy is an extension of medical practice. But we have to contain it," said noted bioethicist the Rev. Richard McCormick, S. J., author of *How Brave a New World?*, "so that it does not lead to germ-line enhancement and eugenic engineering. Scientists are running from the latter two like the plague. I hope common sense would prevail in not attempting to do these experiments. If not, there will have to be government controls."

Leroy Walters, director of bioethics at the Kennedy Institute for the Study of Human Reproduction and Bioethics at Georgetown University and chair of the NIH human gene therapy working group, sees a role for germ cell therapy. "If a way could be devised to carry new genetic material to egg cells or cells that produce sperm, in a predictable, safe, effective way so that the gene would be inserted into the proper cells and would be expressed in the correct way, then it would seem that there would be no ethical objection to try to rid the genetic disease within a given family. Some families would obviously decide the risks are too great." However, as long as the genetic disease was a serious one, and as long as the decision to undergo the therapy was fully informed and freely made, he believes such therapy would be ethically acceptable.

Jonathan Moreno, an ethicist at the Hastings Center, a bioethical think tank, sees more problems with the questions of access, equity and economics related to germ cell therapy than he does with the therapy itself. "I don't have any problems with eliminating certain life-threatening genetic diseases," said Moreno. "I am more concerned with the economics: Access to the elimination of genetic disease will be quite expensive for a long time. People won't have access. And let's go further and ask: What if we were able to manipulate genes for intellectual abilities—it would be hard for black people to have access to it" because of the proportionally large number of blacks who are economically deprived.

Is the Frankenstein myth just that? Do we need to worry about the malevolent scientist who decides that brown eyes are a "bad" genetic trait, or brown skin, or left-handedness? According to Eric Juengst, adjunct lecturer in the division of medical ethics at the University of California at San Francisco, "even more ominous than malevolence is going to be the inertia and drift of broad social forces that will lead us into making mistakes. One place where we are making improvements [now] is in human growth hormone, producing the hormone through recombinant DNA in bacteria and using it to treat hormone deficiencies. The problem is: Who gets it? Those with pituitary dwarfism? How about using it on kids who are marginally short?"

None of these questions is as obscure, futuristic or trivial as it may at first seem. These are all issues that will have to be seriously considered and dealt with. But unlike the situation we now face in the treatment of neonates or in organ transplantation (where we have stampeded into the future and are now discovering that it may be too late to reverse certain trends), the specialty of gene therapy is not yet even in its infancy. Now is the time to ask the questions, and make the decisions, about what kinds of therapies we want to allow and who we want to have controlling these technologies. And if we don't deal with these questions now, we may awaken a decade from now, like a collective Rip Van Winkle, and find that we don't like the world in which we are living very much.

II.
NEW CONCEPTIONS

CHAPTER 3

The Fruitless Quest

Pregnancy was on both Robin and Arthur's minds when they were married in January 1966: It was something they did not want Robin to be. She was nineteen and beginning her junior year of college. He was a self-described "dirty old man" of twenty-four, earning a living stacking cartons of shoes. Unlike many young couples of that era, Robin and Art hadn't spent a lot of time making plans for their future life, talking about having a family. "To tell you the truth, our approach before we got married was to have fun, enjoy each other and plan for the wedding," Art recalled nineteen years later.

Robin began using the then still revolutionary birth control pills shortly before her marriage. She finished college, went on to a career as an elementary school teacher and completed her master's degree. "I think it was assumed that someday we'd have a family," she said, sitting on the sofa beside her husband.

"She may have assumed it," Art said, laughing quietly.

But after Robin had been teaching for about seven years, and Art had worked his way up from stacking cartons of shoes in a shoe store to a successful career as a stockbroker, Robin decided it was time to have a family. That she and Art had managed to avoid getting pregnant for seven years didn't set off any alarms in their heads. While they, like most young people, assumed that getting pregnant was as natural as going to a drive-in movie, they had been careful, and after going off the pill because she developed phlebitis, Robin had faithfully and carefully used a diaphragm. So when she stopped using birth control methods, she assumed she'd become pregnant almost immediately. "After about eight months or so I still was not pregnant. I went to the family doctor and he recommended a gynecologist. I went to see that doctor and of course I was young and healthy and he told me to come back in six months.

Neither Robin nor Art was particularly concerned at that point. Art was sent to New York Hospital–Cornell Medical Center for a sperm count, which he still remembered good-humoredly. The physician who did the testing was "down in the basement of Cornell University hospital. He was busy counting somebody's sperm and came up with forty-eight and I heard him say, 'That'll never make it.' He said mine were jumping like crazy, and I said, 'Thank you very much, doctor,' and that was that."

"I started to use the temperature chart and in about six or seven more months I was pregnant," Robin said. What initial unspoken concerns she and Art may have had were quickly forgotten. The gynecologist wasn't at all concerned because Robin had gotten pregnant within about a year of first trying. In addition, the pregnancy seemed to progress uneventfully. "I kept working and everything seemed fine," Robin recalled. "There was some initial spotting, but no real problems, no reason to put me in bed, no reason for me to stop working." Art recalled that Robin may have been given some "pills" to prevent miscarriage, but she had no recollection of taking anything other than vitamins. "Unfortunately, I wasn't wise enough to get the records from that doctor. We were still kids," she explained. "Anyway, I got into the fourth month and I started having terrible cramping, terrible pain, and I lost the fetus in the toilet bowl. It was quite dreadful. We weren't wise enough either to bring the fetus with us to the hospital. It was a difficult moment," Robin said, in her understated, carefully controlled way.

"So because we didn't have a fetus and because there was nothing to be seen, no doctor could make any conclusion as to why this pregnancy didn't take," Art said.

"It was just miscarry, go home, wait a bit and start over," Robin said. "I think outwardly I fared very well. Inwardly? I didn't grieve. I didn't go into a shell. I didn't have trouble dealing with friends who were becoming pregnant, just a little pang. But I just got out the temperature chart and started again. And about six or seven months later, this would be August of 1973, I was pregnant again."

By Thanksgiving day, Robin was in the fifth month of her pregnancy and everything seemed to be going right. She was visibly pregnant, wearing maternity clothes and thinking about names for the baby. There was no staining this time, no hint that anything might be wrong. Robin had even felt the fetus move for the first time. Thus, nothing prepared her for what happened that afternoon as she was lying on her parents' bed, taking a nap after an enormous family Thanksgiving dinner. Awakening to find herself lying in a puddle of liquid, Robin recalled thinking "I'd urinated all over myself. I didn't know what was happening," she said, having no reason to suspect that her amniotic sac had, at best, begun leaking. Inexplicably, "the doctor said it may or may not be a problem. He said to stay home and rest. I never even got to see him," Robin said, shaking her head in disbelief. "You get smart in your old age. The doctor says, 'Stay home and rest, it's probably nothing,' in those days you stayed home and rested because at that time you thought the doctors knew everything."

But two days later, as she was sitting at her own kitchen table talking to her mother, who was visiting Robin while Robin was baby-sitting for a three-year-old nephew, she "felt just a swelling in the vaginal area and went to the bathroom and there were two little feet sticking out. I said, 'Ma, we have to go to the hospital now.' We used some towels for packing. Thankfully, someone was there. And that was my second miscarriage. They brought me to the hospital in a taxi, they gave me medication to induce labor. I went through about eight hours of labor to deliver the dead fetus." The fetus was superficially examined, but no autopsy was performed. There was no apparent reason for the miscarriage. All the obstetrician could suggest was that Robin might have an incompetent cervix, and that if she became pregnant again he would place stitches in the cervix in an attempt to keep her from miscarrying. "This time I was devastated and this time I said, 'Okay, that's it, I'm not going through this anymore.' The second time was a lot more difficult. I still sometimes see what I saw when I went to the bathroom. It just comes as a flash. It gives me the chills and makes me very sad," Robin said, obviously struggling to retain her composure.

"I felt very bad," Art said wistfully. "I remember in the hospital I had to call up everybody and the tears were just flowing. There was no warning. The first time there was warning. With staining, you know it may happen. But this time, nothing. We had been pleased as punch, everything had been just fine. We were sitting there at the dinner table and she was lying down and her water just broke. It's not that we said we wouldn't try again," Art recalled, "but we lost our enthusiasm."

"I went back on birth control, went back to teaching, and as the years went on, each year there was a little more money, we got to travel, indulge ourselves. If we talked about having a baby, it was to say we'd talk about it another time," Robin said. At that point, as she recalled it, neither she nor Art was feeling under any compulsion to have a child. She spent her entire working week surrounded by young children, and he was busy with his job.

So for seven years Robin used her diaphragm and the subject of babies was forgotten, "until I was about thirty-four and a half years old and the biological clock started to tick and I got that compelling urge to be a mother. At that time that was it, this is what I wanted. It was time, we had no more time, I couldn't wait any longer to decide what I might do. I also must say," she added, "that financially we were in the best situation we'd ever been in. So if I left teaching, and we had to give up my salary, I might have to sacrifice something, but it wouldn't be terrible. I just had this compelling urge. And I don't know if I ever told you this," she said to Art, "but I went in to the family doctor and here I am, thirty-four and a half, and I go through the whole physical and I say to him, 'Do you think I'm too old to have a child?' In essence, am I in physically good condition, can I consider this craziness? And he thought it was terrific, absolutely terrific, and he then recommended the first doctor in the second quest," an obstetrician associated with Mount Sinai Medical Center in Manhattan. "I remember speaking with him on the phone from the doctor's office. The family doctor was so excited about this, he called then and put me on. We were about to leave for Mexico so the OB said, 'Go ahead on your trip and have a good time.' "

When the couple returned from vacation they again began trying to conceive. "But six months later I'm not pregnant and he [the new obstetrician] doesn't want to wait a year because of our age, and he starts testing." And so Robin and Art began the rounds of consultations with physicians, examinations and tests that often become the central focus of the lives of couples with fertility problems. The desire to have a child becomes an obsession: The more they are told they cannot conceive, or carry a

73

child to term, the more they feel compelled to do so. There is always one more thing to try, one more physician who may have the answer. Art had his sperm tested for a second time, and it was again pronounced normal. Then the couple had to suffer through the indignity of postcoital exams, which involve having intercourse and then rushing to the physician's office so he can take a smear for microscopic examination. Next came the hysterosalpingogram, a dye-injection X-ray of the fallopian tubes. The final thing, Robin said, was a laparoscopy, a surgical procedure, under general anesthesia, in which an incision is made in the abdomen and a flexible scope is inserted in order to allow an examination of the fallopian tubes. When all of that was completed, Robin recalled, the doctor said, " 'I have no explanation for you. There is no reason that I can see why you are not becoming pregnant. I'm stifled, I'm stymied, and I would like to refer you to [an infertility specialist on staff at Mount Sinai].' "

The couple's records were transferred to the new physician, who studied the records, ordered a few additional tests and, Robin said, told her and Art that " 'ten percent of infertile couples have unexplained infertility, and I would put you in that category. We have no explanation for you, but have you ever heard of in vitro fertilization?' My husband hadn't heard of in vitro fertilization, but in the summer school vacation I watched all the morning programs so I had heard of in vitro fertilization, but we had to explain to Art what this was all about."

In vitro fertilization was then, and still is, the final option for infertile couples desperate to have their "own" child. Ova, or eggs, are surgically removed from the woman's ovary, fertilized in a laboratory dish—in vitro, or "in glass"—with the husband's sperm, and then placed in the woman's uterus. Despite the fact that advocates of the technique note that in mid-1985 an in vitro baby was born each day somewhere in the world, the technique offers far more hope than pregnancy. At even the best centers, such as that at Eastern Virginia Medical School in Norfolk, Virginia, researchers are lucky to claim a success rate as high as 20 percent, compared with nature's 25 to 30 percent. And at the time Art and Robin were considering entering the brand-new program at Mount Sinai, it was only six months after the birth of Elizabeth Carr, America's first in vitro baby, in Norfolk, and the Mount Sinai program had barely begun.

But as Robin explained, "We wanted a child and were being told that we might never be able to have one, would we consider this? We had to think about it several months. I called up my other obstetrician and he said, 'I wouldn't rush into it, think about it.' We thought about it several months, maybe longer. Then we filled out forms and they said they'd accept us into the program. Originally the concept was not to work with cases of anyone who was over thirty-five. But they accepted us anyway. When we were accepted they wrote us a letter saying they were reevaluating the program and they weren't taking any more patients. Then maybe another six or eight months passed before they said fine, they were ready to take us when we were ready to come in. Then it was at least six or eight months before we got going. And in the meantime, there we are still trying, the thermometer, the whole bit. It was a real horror."

While the idea of trying to get pregnant may sound like fun, many couples going through it know it isn't. As Art described it, "Sex takes place on the five days of greatest fertility and then the rest of the month you forget about it because you have to be ready to perform on those five days. It's really very tough. It was certainly more fun with the diaphragm. But," he added, philosophically, "it certainly wasn't the optimum situation, but we've gone through a lot of things that were tough and this was just one of them."

The in vitro experience was to be another one of those "things that were tough." Art said that they understood, going into the program, that at best it was a "crapshoot, a ten-percent chance, Last Chance Cafe."

"Not even ten percent, five percent," Robin said, interrupting her husband. "We knew we were taking a gamble. But you do it because it's offered to you, it's an opportunity, it's part of the program of becoming pregnant, and we felt that maybe it would work for us—we'd be the lucky ones who beat the odds. If you don't think you're going to beat the odds you don't do this. You really have to believe it's going to work."

"We had a really good attitude going into it too," Art said. "Got gold stars." The couple's records were reviewed once again, there was an educational session that Robin calls "egg class," but there was very little in the way of further testing, probably because of all the screening and testing results that already filled the couple's voluminous medical file. Robin was relieved not to have to repeat all the testing, but the absence of one kind of testing disturbed her. A year later she was still unable to understand why there had been no psychological screening or counseling offered as a formal part of the program.

"No one ever screened us," she said. "We screened ourselves and felt that we could handle it. But there was no psychological counseling. There were some medical interviews and then they put you on the calendar. So in August of 1984 I started the program. I started with the daily monitoring of blood. Every day, starting with day five [of the menstrual cycle]. Then you start taking Pergonal and Clomid [to stimulate ova production and regulate the cycle]. Every day I'd go in on the train with my husband to Mount Sinai and all of his train friends couldn't imagine why I was going in. And I had to be there at eight-thirty in the morning because they had to have the results so at two in the afternoon they could tell me how much medication to take, meaning the Pergonal. That's about ten days of doing that, starting with day five, until a certain point in your cycle. I took

Clomid in pill form and injections of Pergonal," which Art, a former army medic, administered. "Then just about on day twelve they give you a shot of Pergonal and within thirty-six hours or so they know that you're going to ovulate and that's when they want you on the operating table."

"We established a new procedure for them: how to set up in the operating room without being scheduled for an operating room," Art said.

"The program was very young, and one did at times feel somewhat like a guinea pig," Robin continued. "But you forget about that because it's a chance." And at the end of the second week of the first attempt, the real chance came. "I had just gotten home from the hospital and was about ready to eat and the nurse who was in the program at the time calls me up and says, 'Have you eaten anything?' I said, 'I've just put one spoonful in my mouth.' 'Spit it out!' We drove back into the city, this was on a Friday night. I undressed in the operating room because they had to take me quickly or they'd lose the eggs. That first time they were a little off in the timing," Robin said, but they recovered two "good" eggs. The eggs were then "washed" and allowed to mature for about another six hours—as they would naturally when traveling down the fallopian tubes—before Art's sperm were placed in the petri dish. One of the two eggs fertilized and began to cleave, or divide. "Then two days later you come in and they've got the little pipette. The transfer is done in one of the hospital operating rooms, you're just on your back for four hours and then you go home and you wait for two more weeks.

"I went in as soon as it was possible to get the blood test," Robin continued, "and we got the results and they were negative. And it was very, very, very hard. Everything went textbook, everything went perfectly, and we didn't beat the odds. Nothing happened."

77

"So," Art said, "we said, 'Doctor, what do you think we should do?' "

"And the team agreed I responded so well, everything was terrific and we knew going in that, based on the experience of other couples who had been through the program in other places, that it takes more than one time," Robin said. "So you're resigned to the fact that it's more than one time. You also have to start wondering, 'Well, how many times can I go through this?' and you have to start to set limits."

"Then the doctors say, 'It's a crapshoot, and the more times you go, the better your odds.' But it's still the same five to ten percent each time," Art said, laughing softly, "but keep you keep trying."

"You're blue," Robin said, "and you're sad and you're upset, but then you start gearing up for the next one and then you get high again." So in November 1985 the second in vitro attempt began.

"And the second time there are no problems," Art said, "and the thirty days go faster. The first time you're going through it it seems to creep. But the second time, you realize each step is the building block for the next. You need to go through each step and some people drop out at each step. But we knew we were going to be a textbook case and the time just flew," he said, snapping his fingers for emphasis. Not only did the time fly, but the second laparoscopy yielded seven eggs, and six were fertilized. The director of the program called Robin at home, the evening before the implantation, and, as she remembered it a year later, "he was going crazy. He said, 'Oh my God, six eggs, and I think we're going to put them all back in. See you tomorrow, and of course you could have a multiple birth,' but we knew that from the start.

"So the next morning I'm up in the operating room with one of the OB-GYNs from the team and he said the director of the team wanted to speak to me. The director said that, of the six eggs, four just stopped cleaving at the same stage—they all were cleaving the day before. He said he had never seen anything like this in humans. They only had two instead of six, but that was okay. So they transferred two. And we waited. And we wondered what was this crazy thing where they all stopped cleaving at the same time. And we were talking about how we were going to name the kids, you play that game, you have to play that game. And again I wasn't pregnant," Robin said, sounding as depressed as she had obviously been. "And now Art and I had to sit down and say, 'This is crazy. What are we going to do? How many more times will we go through this?' And before we went to see the director, we kind of made a decision: If they wanted to try one more time, we'd go one more time. And then, no matter what they say, they're not getting me back."

Robin continued: "After the problem with the cleavage, the director of the program said, 'You know, you've tried so hard, you've been through so much, I would like you to go for a genetic workup. Let's see what we can find out. Chances are we can't find anything, because we can only detect so much, but let's see what we can find out. I'd like you to do that, maybe we can come up with a genetic reason.' He was hooked on finding a genetic reason. Maybe it didn't happen to every egg, but maybe that's the problem. So they did the genetic workup, and still couldn't find anything, they couldn't find anything but he still believed it was a genetic problem. He said, 'Your odds may not be as good as someone else's, but you've still got a shot.'

"And we went one more time, in February of '85," Robin continued. "And we go through the whole thing again, the monitoring, the going to the hospital, and everything is perfect. We go in and we have another laparoscopy. And we got eight eggs, and six of them look terrific, and we go home and the nurse calls and says, 'Everything is terrific. We have at least five or six terrific eggs to transfer and we're thrilled.' It's our last chance and maybe God's going to be good to us, this is when you say, 'Maybe God's going to be good to us.'

"Then it's a Saturday morning and we go into the hospital and go to admitting and there's a note from [a doctor on the team] to call her at home. All of the eggs stopped cleaving, and there we were in the hospital with no place to go. They had been unable to reach us because we had left very early and we were always concerned about traffic on the expressway and would we get there in time because the eggs must go in at a certain point—and we had no eggs. . . ."

"And there we are, sitting in the admitting office all by our lonesome, and we'd been told it was over," Art said.

"Crying," his wife continued, "because we knew that this was it, the Last Chance Corral."

"It was very sad, it was so sad," Art said, uncharacteristically quietly. "Ask us how we pulled our pants up and moved up on that one. . . ."

"The next day we took a drive out to wine country, in February," Robin said.

"We drove to Orient Point, which is about two and a half hours from here, the end of the island," Art continued. "We figured we wanted to see the end of the world. . . ."

"To throw ourselves off into the ocean," Robin said. "I remember being very quiet. I cried a lot. This really was the last chance. I would not go through this again. And still not having an answer was very, very tough."

"So we thought about adopting, and we're working for an independent adoption," Art said.

"And I was recommended to another doctor," Robin said, "and he read my medical records and saw some loopholes, some things that we had never done."

"He says there are always answers," said Art, who is more desperate for answers than he is for a child.

"He does not believe there are no answers," Robin said. "We're working with him and he sees some things. I have chlamydia. How long I've had chlamydia I don't know. And we've discovered that Art has an antibody problem. So we're working with this new doctor and we could end up having an adopted baby and another baby."

How did a simple desire to have children turn into a compulsion, a compulsion that, prior to financing a private adoption, had cost Art and Robin about $25,000?

"The more they tell you they don't know, or the more they tell you no, it's just like with a child, the more you want it, the more you feel it, the more you taste it, the more when you see a child you'd like to hold it and grab it and take care of it," Robin said. "It just builds, it just keeps building as you go on and on and on. I have to have closure. I would like an answer. Tell me it's because my eyes are blue. Give me a reason. I have to have a reason. I just am not satisfied. I'm a very obsessive, compulsive person, and I can't deal with not having an explanation, and there has been no closure. And it bothers me."

"I've always wanted to be a father by the time I was forty," Art said, smiling.

"Art's father was forty when he [Art] was born and we've talked about this, how did he feel about having a father that was older than everybody else's father," Robin explained. "He had no problem with it, and I don't feel thirty-nine, but it does become a compulsion in the quest to give me an answer, tell me something. I can't believe there isn't an answer."

Art continued: "It's also another thing: We've been very lucky, and acquired a lot of things in our life, and there comes a time when you say, 'I'd like to have a child.' And it came five years ago. And here we've been denied that benefit, or satisfaction. Does it become a compulsion? Yeah, I guess so. To the degree that why can't I get satisfaction in this area when I've gotten it everywhere else. Nothing's been denied to me prior to this, why should this be the situation where I'm not finding satisfaction? And on that basis we get crazy too. It's not a question of 'Is God punishing us?' "

"I got past that," Robin said, "but you do a lot of 'why me?' throughout this whole procedure."

"But the God curse, that whole business, we don't stay up at night brooding about it," Art said. "But when people who are on welfare can have kids and we can't. . . ." He slowly shook his head from side to side.

Robin said she was unhappy about the in vitro process, in part because no matter how informed the consent, the desperate will believe what they want to believe. "You're told what it is. You read all the paperwork, you read all the forms. There are a whole lot of documents that you go through. But if you believed what was on the paper you wouldn't do it. You don't believe it. You say it isn't going to be that way with me . . . if you believed all of that you couldn't do it, that this could happen and that could happen and this could happen. They tell you, 'You realize the success rate is very low,' and you ask if they've had successes and they hadn't. But if you believed it was that bad, you wouldn't do it. I believe in vitro serves a purpose, but was it for me? I don't know. But it was a hope when we had no hope."

"And we took it," Art said, "we definitely wanted to take it. We also knew, going in—and our attitude happened to be much better than it is now—going in we accepted the odds, we thought we'd be winners, but we knew we really didn't have that much of a chance, and when it didn't happen, as much as we were disappointed, we were still anxious to do it again. There weren't second thoughts about doing it again. We were ready to do it again, and my wife said, 'How long would it be before we take our second chance?' So they said, 'Take one month off to clean out your system and you're welcome to come back again.' And the second time, it went from seven eggs to one or two, and we weren't ready to back off. You can get caught into almost a gambler's syndrome. It didn't occur to us, but I can see where it can happen, people say I know I'm going to be a winner. Let me pull the machine one more time and I'll come up with three gold bars, I'll hit the jackpot. Maybe if you can afford to do it you'll go broke doing it."

What of the $25,000 spent on a gamble?

"What dollars are important when you're trying to bring life into the world? I'm not being factitious," Art said, "it depends on your value system. Let me ask you a question. A woman can go out and buy a mink coat for $5000. She can buy a lynx coat for $7500, $8000. She can buy a fisher for $15,000 or $16,000 and she can go out and get a sable for $25,000 to $35,000. Depending upon how she hits her husband or boyfriend over the head, there'll be a certain expense. Now here's a situation that's a joint effort between husband and wife and it involves the expression of love, and the fruition of the family and all the traditional values: So what expenditure is reasonable?"

"Everybody does draw a line," Robin said. "I haven't drawn a line except to say to myself and Art that I'm going to be forty years old in May and that's it. I'd like to have an answer. But . . ."

"I called my lawyer and said, 'Get me a kid. Don't buy me a kid. The legitimate way, get me a kid.' "

Will they be satisfied with an adopted child?

"I wonder," Robin said. "Loving a child doesn't satisfy my trouble with not having an answer. . . ."

CHAPTER 4

Getting Pregnant in the Eighties

Less than twenty years ago there was very little that medical science could offer the 2.5 million American couples who, like Art and Robin, were unable to conceive or carry a pregnancy to term. There were physicians who handled such cases, but they were closer in spirit to witch doctors than to today's top infertility specialists, who are likely to be embryologists or endocrinologists. In most cases, these "specialists" could only narrow down the possible causes of infertility by counting and testing the male's sperm and determining if the woman was ovulating properly and if her fallopian tubes were clear. But if her tubes were blocked, there was little physicians could do. Microsurgery was still barely in its infancy, and repairing damaged tubes was far beyond the skill of all but the smallest handful of gynecological surgeons. If a woman had repeated miscarriages, her obstetrician could either stitch up her cervix and put her to bed for nine months or offer her the "wonder drug" DES, which we have since learned did little to prevent miscarriage but greatly increased the risk of uterine cancer in the daughters of women who used it during pregnancy.

Because we now take in vitro fertilization relatively for

granted, we tend to forget that the world's first in vitro baby, Louise Brown, was born just eight years ago, on July 25, 1978. It is now estimated that there are more than 700 infants conceived this way around the world, and another being born each day. We have also witnessed the birth of the first embryo-transfer baby, conceived in one woman and carried to term in the uterus of another; we have seen "surrogate mothers" appear on network talk shows; and we have seen ethicists and even governments attempt to grapple with the farfetched question—given the fact that twenty-four-week fetuses have no rights if their mothers want them aborted—of whether a frozen embryo has "rights" after both its parents are killed.

Unfortunately, media fascination with and coverage of such peripheral issues as whether the frozen embryo of a deceased wealthy couple will inherit their estate should that embryo be thawed and carried to term in an adoptive mother's uterus distract us from some of the real hard choices that face us in the field of reproductive technology. Because the government is not funding research in embryo transfer, in vitro fertilization or any of the other more arcane areas of infertility treatment, it is easy for society as a whole to ignore these issues, leaving privately funded institutions and individuals to carry on their work unchallenged by anyone other than right-to-life advocates and bioethicists. But the fact that this research is being privately funded on either a pay-as-you-go or a venture capital basis does not mean that it is free to society, nor that we should fail to ask the same kind of questions about its propriety that we would ask about any government-funded research.

Before discussing the funding of this research, we should briefly examine these new methods of achieving pregnancy and consider some of the ethical questions they raise.

Artificial insemination—which results in an estimated 10,000 to 20,000 pregnancies a year—is the oldest of these conception technologies, and the one with which society seems to be the most comfortable. Used successfully in agriculture for so long that there are numerous generations of cows who have never seen a bull, human artificial insemination involves either the collection and freezing of donor sperm or the direct donation of fresh sperm. While some couples, particularly some males, are uncomfortable with the idea of the wife being impregnated with sperm donated by another man, the use of artificial insemination (AI) gives couples in which the husband fails to produce sperm or has an extremely low sperm count a chance to experience a normal pregnancy and have a child. AI may also be used in cases of infertility caused by a chemical or mechanical abnormality in the cervical area that prevents sperm from entering the uterus. In such cases the wife can be artificially inseminated with her husband's sperm, and can then go on to bear a child that is genetically hers and her husband's. In more typical AI cases, the child born of the process is the genetic progeny of the woman and the sperm donor, who is usually unknown to either husband or wife.

Like many of the questions raised by the use of the fertilization technologies, the hard choices posed by AI tend to be legal more often than ethical, with variation from state to state over the legitimacy and fatherhood of children conceived with donor sperm. There are also, of course, a number of "what if's" concerning ethical or moral issues surrounding AI. What if, for instance, a large number of women decide they would be better off living without men and choose to bear children conceived via AI? What if lesbian couples use AI to have children? What if a woman who wants children when her husband doesn't decides to become pregnant with the aid of AI? What if AI is used by couples for sex selection, to ensure that they will have either the male or the female child they desire? What, in general, would expanded use of AI do to the natural order of things? All of these are intensely personal questions for the individuals involved.

86

Were they to be raised widely, however, they would pose questions about the future of the family as we know it, and hence about the structure and survival of our society in its present form. At least that's the concern of those who spend their careers considering such questions. But at this point, it is probably safe to leave those particular worries to the professional ethicists and moral theologians to debate while the public concentrates on more pressing ethical and financial hard choices.

There are, however, some other considerations. AI can be used for selective breeding in humans, just as it is in cattle. In addition to the very real concern about the use of AI as a way to guarantee the birth of a child of a given sex, we have the Repository for Germinal Choice, Robert K. Graham's "Nobel Prize sperm bank," to consider. The California septuagenarian, who had already given the world shatter-proof eye glasses, decided that what the world still needed was a sperm bank filled with the deposits of Nobel Prize winners and others of presumably superior genetic endowment, including Olympic medalists. The only publicly identified depositor at Graham's bank was William B. Shockley, who won a Nobel for inventing the transistor, but is far better known for his publicly espoused view that the Negroid race is genetically inferior intellectually to the Caucasian race. Graham contends that his effort is in no way racist but is simply dedicated to providing the world with a greater number of intellectually and physically outstanding individuals.

Like artificial insemination, in vitro fertilization has been opposed by the Catholic Church on the grounds of its artificiality. But its use, per se, does not trouble many bioethicists. If used as intended, this fertilization technique is really no more than a gynecological plumbing trick, allowing women with blocked or missing fallopian tubes to bear children. Despite the fact that the public refers to infants conceived by the in vitro process as "test tube" babies, these infants are no different from those conceived during sexual intercourse. As Art and Robin, and the thousands of other couples undergoing in vitro fertilization, learned, at its most basic level, the process involves nothing more than removing ripe ova from the woman, placing them in a culture medium with the husband's sperm and then placing the fertilized ova in the woman's uterus where, it is hoped, at least one will continue to develop and be carried to term. These are hardly the babies of Huxley's *Brave New World.* And about the only persons objecting to the use of the in vitro process are those rabid right-to-lifers who view the fertilized ovum as a person, with all the rights of a term infant, or an adult for that matter, and worry that less than perfect fertilized ova are being flushed down laboratory sinks. They are, of course, correct. The in vitro programs here and abroad are destroying those embryos that appear grossly abnormal. But what do the right-to-life advocates think happens in nature? According to one major study, fertilization occurs only about 85 percent of the time when ova are naturally exposed to sperm. Of those ova that are fertilized, it is estimated that only 50 percent survive to the second week of development. So half of all ova either fail to attach to the uterine wall or are flushed from the uterus because of some problem in the uterine environment or because some abnormality in the embryo triggers the rejection process. This study, cited by the since disbanded H.E.W. Ethics Advisory Board in its report on in vitro fertilization and embryo transfer, concludes that "only 37 percent of human zygotes survive to be delivered subsequently as live infants. Statistical surveys of the length of time generally required to establish a pregnancy seem to lend support to these estimates." If those embryo losses occur naturally, one then has to ask why shouldn't the in vitro effort proceed if the main ethical argument against it is that it leads to the "killing" of imperfect embryos? After all, those same imperfect embryos would be killed in nature.

No, the hard choices raised by in vitro fertilization really have very little to do with the fertilization method itself. Rather, they concern the manner in which ova fertilized in the laboratory are subsequently carried to term. And so we come to the more bizarre and far more troubling of what might be called reproductive configurations.

Among these is embryo freezing, which has resulted in the birth of at least one human infant and countless mice and cattle. This technique involves harvesting as many ripe ova as possible from a woman, fertilizing the ova, allowing their development to the six- or eight-cell stage and then freezing the resulting embryos for future gestation. While researchers obviously do not know the long-term implications of human embryo freezing, the technique has been used for years to preserve specific gene lines in animals. The Jackson Laboratory in Bar Harbor, Maine, the world's largest supplier of genetically "pure" mice to research laboratories around the world, routinely freezes embryos to preserve the hundreds of strains of mice bred for their particular genetic defects. The embryos of hairless mice, blind mice, diabetic mice, spastic mice, fat mice and thin mice, and mice prone to all varieties of tumor are frozen to preserve the various strains in the event that disease or accidental crossbreeding destroys them. Thus far at least one strain that was accidentally lost has been continued through the use of the frozen embryos. Even assuming that the freezing and thawing process does not damage human embryos, the use of the process raises the specter of infertile couples purchasing frozen embryos for implantation in either the female purchaser or the rented uterus of a surrogate mother. In this area, like many others related to the new conceptions, the technology has long ago outstripped the law and ethics, and a chain of frozen embryo franchises could be part of the landscape long before we consider the implications of the technology.

Another of the new configurations is donor embryo transfer, a process by which woman A agrees, presumably for a fee, either to be artificially inseminated with the sperm of the husband of woman B or to have her ova harvested for in vitro fertilization by woman B's husband's sperm. The fertilized ova are then either flushed from woman A's donor's reproductive tract or taken from the lab dish, and implanted in woman B's uterus. Perfected by Dr. John Buster of the University of Southern California—and financed by a group of venture capitalists who want to patent the medical technique—the conception configuration in which the ovum donor is artificially inseminated and then "flushed" had resulted in the delivery of two infants by late 1985. On first consideration it seems theoretically little different from sperm donation. But shortly after the announcement of his program's first success, Buster said during a lengthy interview that embryo transfer involves "a complete turnaround in how people relate to each other. It involves exchanging commodities that no one has ever exchanged before, and the ethics and morality and legal aspects of this thing are just not worked out yet because we've never done this before. . . . There's no question it's a biologically reasonable thing to do," Buster said. "There's no question that families can really support each other in various ways by doing this when otherwise there would be no support. And finally, it's very apparent that women who aren't even related to each other can support each other knowing that an egg goes out there some place and becomes a baby and a family will exist because of that gift that someone gave. It's very, very basic stuff, and it's going to take us all a while to sort out our feelings about this."

There are other important questions, too. During the interview Buster was asked if the potential donors were screened for physical appearance, as well as for health, intelligence and personality stability. "I wouldn't say it publicly that we dropped some because they weren't very attractive, but we did," he replied. Does that kind of selection process place an embryo transfer program on a par with a sperm bank that chooses its donors based on their IQ or ability to run the 440? And what happens if a donor mother later decides she wants the child that is genetically 50 percent hers? What if she decides, if she has been impregnated by artificial insemination, that she does not want her ova harvested? Is this situation analogous to an adoption procedure in which a woman signs away rights to her baby? If it is analogous, is it the same as the situation before or after the birth of the baby that is going to be given up?

From in vitro embryo transfer we "progress" to in vitro embryo transfer involving a surrogate mother. First performed once in 1985, this conceptual ménage à trois is a "rent-a-womb" arrangement, whereby woman A, who is presumably unable to carry a pregnancy to term, and her husband conceive through the in vitro process. But instead of implanting this genetic progeny of woman A and her husband in woman A's uterus, the in vitro specialist implants the fertilized ova in the uterus of woman B, who has agreed to carry the pregnancy to term and then surrender the infant to woman A and her husband. When this technique was first used, at Mount Sinai Medical Center in Cleveland, the case was described to the press as an exceptional one and one that was reviewed carefully by the hospital's institutional review board. In that case, woman B was described as a close friend of woman A who was simply trying to help woman A and her husband have a child. But this technique could be established on a strictly cash-and-carry basis. And that's where it gets particularly troubling. Will the in vitro–surrogate configuration provide a means for professional women to have babies without ever having a baby? Will two-professional couples simply provide rent-a-womb brokers with their genetic material (in the form of ovum and sperm) and return nine months later to pick up their babies? No fuss, no muss, no maternity wardrobe, no career interruption other than perhaps a three- to six-week "maternity leave" to get the baby established at home with the nanny. Admittedly, this is a relatively farfetched scenario. But the very concept of in vitro–surrogate motherhood was considered farfetched less than a year before the birth of the first baby conceived and carried to term using the configuration. And who would have guessed, in 1977, that by 1985 there would be in vitro fertilization clinics in most American cities of any size, and there would be an in vitro baby born every day somewhere in the world. In these days of swiftly proliferating medical "miracles" it does not take long for yesterday's "farfetched" idea or technique to become today's commonplace reality.

After all, the public hadn't even heard of surrogate motherhood prior to the 1980s, and halfway through the decade that arrangement is taken for granted, although considered "unusual" at best. But there have reportedly been hundreds of women who, for fees around $10,000, have agreed to be artificially inseminated with the sperm of a man whose wife is infertile in order that the infertile couple might have a baby that is at least half theirs genetically. The legality of such arrangements is questionable at best in a number of states and nonexistent in others. To paraphrase the title of a play and movie dealing with another hard choice: "Whose child is it anyway?" Is the child born of the surrogate mother her child, to be given up for adoption? Is it the child of the couple who arranged for its birth? Does the infertile woman, whose husband's sperm fertilized the surrogate, have any legal claim to the infant? And what do you tell your surrogate baby when it is old enough to ask the questions adoptive children eventually ask?

There are three basic questions that are posed by the very existence of these alternative forms of conception and gestation: Should they be available? What are their costs? And should their development and use be regulated?

The answer to the first question really depends upon our answer to the second two, for these technologies do exist now, and more are coming on line every year, if not every month. Scientific "advances" cannot be willed away. So what are we going to do with these conception technologies and configurations now that we have them? In vitro fertilization undeniably can be of help to a small fraction of the 2.5 million couples who would like to have children but can't. But if this technology is available, how should it be paid for? It can be argued that it would be obscene for the government to pay for in vitro fertilization attempts, or to fund research into in vitro fertilization, in an overpopulated world. But as in every other area of science, research to improve in vitro techniques has indirect payoffs, providing science with information about conception and embryo development, information that may eventually help to explain, for example, what happens when a normal cell becomes cancerous. There is no question that even if the government and private insurance companies are not paying for this research, it is still costing money and it is still diverting laboratory resources and skilled personnel who could be engaged in more pressing research or health care delivery. But clearly those researchers are right who argue that ending the flow of resources and energy to one scientific endeavor does not in any way guarantee that those resources and energy will end up in any other particular endeavor.

Because we cannot stop research in these areas—or control the sources of funding—and because the desperation of would-be parents is such there would probably be black-market conception technology if use of the technologies was outlawed, perhaps the government should be funding some of this research as a way to regulate it. After all, the most powerful enforcement tool the government science bureaucracy has at this time is its ultimate threat to cut off funding. If it doesn't provide any funding to a given program and that program is in a free-standing institution hat doesn't receive government funds, then what enforcement power does the government have?

But before we consider how to enforce regulations or standards we have to come to a consensus as to what those regulations and standards are or should be. And that is something we are a long way from doing. The first step toward establishing such a consensus would be to reestablish the Ethics Advisory Board within the federal Department of Health and Human Services, something the Reagan administration has refused to do in the mistaken belief that if the government is not involved in making these hard choices they will not be made. Unfortunately, they will be made anyway, but they will be made with an eye to the bottom line on a corporate balance sheet, rather than to the long-term societal impact these conception technologies and configurations may have.

III.
FETAL INTERVENTION

CHAPTER 5

Michael and Nicholas

Between the moment of conception—no matter how that conception is achieved—and the moment of delivery so much can go wrong that it truly is a miracle that so much goes right. At every step in the process of cell differentiation and fetal development, accidents may occur that can result in the birth of a blind, deaf, crippled or retarded infant, or one who is all of those things. A palate may not form properly, causing the baby to be born with a gaping maw instead of a normal mouth. Limb buds may remain just that, resulting in the birth of an infant resembling a seal. An opening between the diaphragm and the chest cavity—a simple diaphragmatic hernia—may result in the movement of intestines into the chest cavity, leaving the lungs without room to develop. A urinary tract blockage that is easy enough to correct in the newborn may destroy the kidneys before birth.

Until the development of prenatal diagnosis, particularly of ultrasonography, women and their obstetricians rarely if ever knew that these potentially devastating anomalies were occurring. Now, however, these imaging technologies have provided a window into the uterus, and parents and physicians alike have a way of knowing when something is dreadfully amiss. Some of these problems are essentially chemical and can now be treated with drugs. Some require interuterine fetal blood transfusions, a feat first attempted successfully about twenty years ago and today a relatively commonplace, albeit hardly risk-free, technique. But other anomalies require surgery to correct, if they can be corrected at all. And before we consider the hard choices posed by fetal surgery, listen to the stories of Michael Skinner and Nicholas Hannan, two of only a few dozen subjects of highly experimental fetal surgery.

Rosa Skinner did not have any premonitions or worries about the fetus she was carrying in January 1981, but because of her "advanced maternal age"—she was forty-one and pregnant with her fourth child—she was scheduled for amniocentesis. She could have had the test conducted close to her San Mateo, California, home. But Dr. Mitchell Golbus of the University of California's Moffitt Hospital in San Francisco had conducted the amnios during two of her previous pregnancies, so she chose to go to him again. The first thing Mrs. Skinner learned on the morning of January 8 was that she was carrying twins. "You're kidding!" she remembered telling the ultrasound technician who was scanning the uterus preparatory to the amniocentesis. The technician wasn't kidding.

And the technician was also serious when she said she thought she saw a mass in the uterus in addition to the twins. Rosa Skinner then had to spend a weekend—until she could be examined by Golbus himself—waiting to find out if she had cancer. When he examined Mrs. Skinner, Golbus couldn't find the mass the technician thought she had spotted. But Golbus was worried by something else he saw, so he had the woman examined by Dr. Roy Filly, the senior ultrasonographer at Moffitt. What the two men found, they explained to Mrs. Skinner, was that the abdomen of one of the two fetuses seemed to be overloaded with fluid. "They said, 'we don't know what causes this,' " the woman recalled,

" 'but the condition of the fetus is so severe that the fetus is going to go into cardiac arrest and you're going to abort both fetuses.' " If the two fetuses were carried to term, the physicians counseled, one might be healthy. "But they said, 'Don't paint the room, don't get the furniture and don't buy baby clothes, because you're going to abort them. It could happen in a week, it could happen in a month.' I asked what I could do and they said the only thing was to observe the fetus with ultrasound."

Through the winter and into the early spring, Rosa Skinner worried and the doctors watched. Then on April 10, when the woman already knew she was carrying a boy and a girl but did not know which one was sick, Roy Filly discovered that the fluid was backing up into the kidneys of the male fetus and its organs were being forced up into the chest cavity, compressing the lungs. During ultrasound examinations "I could see the spine curving out from the pressure," said Mrs. Skinner, who was then told to leave the examination room but not the hospital.

That day, said Rosa Skinner, she was finally told what was really going on. "Dr. Golbus explained for the first time that the boy had the problem and the girl was all right. He said the boy could go into cardiac arrest at any time, that he was under tremendous pressure, and they said the danger right then was to his kidneys. They said the ureters [the tubes connecting the kidneys and bladder] were bigger than an adult's. They said the urine was dangerously building up into the kidneys. He explained it would be a very easy problem to correct in an adult—they'd just put in a catheter and let it drain. He also said the female fetus was in danger, too. Then he said there was something we could do."

And it was then that Rosa Skinner learned how fortuitous it was she had decided to travel to San Francisco and Mitchell Golbus for her amniocentesis. Golbus and Filly were two of the three co-directors of the pioneering fetal treatment program at UCSF, which has been centered on the treatment of hydronephrosis, the condition threatening the male twin. Golbus "explained that he could try to insert a catheter into [the fetal] bladder and empty it into the amniotic sac. It sounded like the perfect thing to do, but he said it had never been done before. Right then my husband and I looked at each other and said it should be done. We decided right then and there. It was a struggle between life and death. Dr. Golbus said, 'You don't have to decide now. Go home and think about it.' He said he had to talk to some people about it and get it cleared. But he said time was of the essence."

That was on April 10. Three days later, Rosa Skinner was lying on an operating table, under mild sedation, tilted at a forty-five-degree angle to increase blood flow to the placenta. She had been given a drug to reduce the chances of her going into premature labor because of the procedure. When the catheter was inserted through her abdomen into the fetus she recalled feeling "this tremendous rush of water, just a whooosh! across my abdomen." She remembers: "Dr. Golbus said it was urine. The baby was so filled up with it it was just like piercing a boil."

While the physicians managed to drain the fluid from the fetus, the instruments they had wouldn't work properly with the cathether designed by surgeon Michael Harrison (the program's third co-director) so the procedure had to be concluded without the installation of a semipermanent drain. "It was disappointing," Rosa Skinner said. "When they wheeled me back into the room they said that they had drained the baby's bladder and that had bought time. I said, 'How about the people who make your needles for amniocentesis? Couldn't you draw something and describe it to them over the phone?' Dr. Golbus said time was of the essence, and he didn't want to get my hopes up, but they'd try. And my husband and I were thinking how sad it would be to see [the fetus] die for something that would be so easy to correct."

The following week, with a sonogram showing the fluid build-ing up again, Golbus told the woman that a firm had agreed to manufacture the necessary equipment. "We were overjoyed," she recalled. "You know how when you go to a funeral after somebody's died and you come home and feel let down? That's how we'd been feeling—like we'd buried him already. Dr. Har-rison explained that there were other possible procedures, all of them tried only on sheep. In theory it would be possible to lift out the fetus and operate, but with twins that would be too com-plicated." So the route once again would be to insert a catheter through Rosa Skinner's abdomen into the fetus to allow the fluid to drain into the amniotic sac.

On April 26 Mrs. Skinner arose alone at dawn to drive to Moffitt, leaving her aircraft mechanic husband, who had been working the graveyard shift, at home asleep. As she made the half-hour drive, what she calls her "great responsibility to the healthy baby" weighed on her mind.

"I wanted another little girl," she said. "I just didn't want to abort a healthy fetus. I couldn't do that if there was only one fetus. But the doctors were giving me a chance—not just a chance to save one baby, because by saving one I was saving the other too."

By 8 A.M. the expectant mother was again lying on the operating table, neither tilted as much nor strapped as she had been the first time. "They told me I mustn't move under any circumstances, and I was even afraid to breathe," she recalled. "I figured if they had the needle in the right place I wasn't going to breathe deep enough to move the needle out. They used a sono-gram machine to guide themselves during the surgery, and I could hear them talking back and forth." The doctors were tak-ing turns trying to get the catheter in the right position. "I could hear them say, 'I'll try it again,' " she said. "Finally when they reached it I heard Dr. Harrison say, 'Okay, it's in place now.' It was really thrilling. I felt the baby move and I said, 'Dr. Harrison, the baby's moving.' He said, 'It's okay. The catheter's in place and the needle's out now.' I started crying. At least he was going to get a chance."

On May 10, 1981, Mother's Day, Michael and Mary Skinner were born five to six weeks premature, a common occurrence for twins.

Mary was completely normal. Michael was not.

Michael was operated on the day after his delivery. His ureters were cut and led outside his body to drain directly into his diaper. At the same time a hernia in his diaphragm was repaired and the organs that had been forced up against his lungs were placed in their proper positions. Three weeks after the surgery the fluid began to build up again in Michael's kidneys. The pediatricians urged a revision of the surgery on the ureters, but Rosa Skinner remembered Michael Harrison telling her, " 'I know this looks very critical. But I don't think there's need for surgery. I think it's going to work itself out. If you want me to operate I will, but I think we should just wait a bit and see how he does.' We felt that if they operated again then he wouldn't live, so we waited. And you know, the next day he started improving."

During his first year Michael Skinner had respiratory difficulties caused by the compression of his lungs in utero. As his mother recalled, Michael had trouble crying. "But I'd let him cry," Mrs. Skinner said, "because I remember my mother saying it was the only way babies could exercise their lungs. So I'd let him cry and I'd cry. And he couldn't nurse, so I rented an electric [breast] pump and I used it every two hours until two A.M. . . . And then I was just so exhausted I had to sleep."

By the time Michael returned to Moffitt at one year for an operation to reconnect his ureters, however, he was chattering away, saying, "Hi there! Hi there!" to anyone who would listen. And at two years he was walking, talking and climbing onto and into every available object, as does any two-year-old. "I didn't make any promises to God," Rosa Skinner said. "I just prayed to God to help me and . . . it's a miracle. Sometimes I just can't believe he's fine now. His kidneys are fine—there's no damage. His heart's fine and his lungs are fine. Everything is fine."

As it was to Rosa Skinner, the very concept of fetal surgery was also unfamiliar to Sara Hannan in 1981. The Colorado housewife was in about the eighteenth week of her second, planned pregnancy when she began to sense that something wasn't quite right with the fetus. "He was very active," she recalled, "and I thought I had an octopus. I could tell he was kind of in pain. He started kicking very early, when the doctor said I shouldn't feel it. He thought I might have twins." Because of that suspicion, the general surgeon who cared for Sara Hannan in the small farming community in which she lived arranged to have a technician with a portable ultrasound unit drive the one hundred fifty miles from Denver on December 15, 1981, to confirm, or rule out, the possibility that the twenty-six-year-old woman was carrying twins. Sara Hannan was unfamiliar with the use of ultrasound and what are to the untrained the confusing images it produces, but as she lay on her back on an examining table, with the technician running the machine's probe over her oiled abdomen, she was frightened by what she saw. "I saw the picture of his head, and I saw the two black pockets of water, and I said to the technician, 'What's that?' She couldn't give me an answer because it wasn't her place [job]."

But the following day the surgeon called the Hannans and told them to be in his office at four the following afternoon. "We were concerned because they stressed that I should come along," said Daniel Hannan, a computer technician. When the couple sat down with the surgeon he explained that the ultrasound had revealed that Sara was carrying a fetus suffering from hydrocephalus, a buildup of fluid in the ventricles of the brain, normally empty chambers, caused by the blockage of the channels that allow the fluid to drain into the body. The buildup of fluid, and consequent swelling of the skull, can compress the brain and cause brain damage before birth. After birth, if a shunt, or drainage tube, is not surgically implanted, the head can continue to swell to enormous proportions, causing severe retardation and eventual death.

The picture painted for the Hannans was a grim one, but their doctor told them he seemed to remember reading something about fetal surgery in the *New England Journal of Medicine* and had arranged for a consultation for the couple the following day at the University of Colorado Medical Center. Setting off for Denver in the predawn December darkness, Sara Hannan remembers thinking, "This had to be happening to somebody else. I didn't understand it, and we were hoping the diagnosis was wrong."

But this time even the technician told the young mother that the diagnosis was correct. "I almost threw up," Sara Hannan said. "I was weak in the knees." Surgeon William Clewell, a member of the University of Colorado's fetal surgery team, told the Hannans that he considered their fetus a good candidate for the experimental surgical procedure first attempted at the university in 1980, and he gave them the weekend to consider their options. Clewell explained that if the prenatal surgery was successful it might stop the swelling in the skull, relieve the pressure on the brain and prevent further brain damage, if any had already occurred. "He explained the different possibilities that there are," Sara Hannan recalled, "either termination or continuation and leave it alone and see how bad it becomes." Clewell explained that normally, if a fetus with hydrocephalus was not aborted, its development would simply be followed closely with ultrasound. Those involved in the care of mother and fetus would then know how much the head was swelling as fluid, and thus pressure, built up inside. They would also be able to gauge how much of the brain was being damaged by the fluid filling the skull. If such a case is diagnosed prior to birth, a cesarean delivery can be planned ahead of time and a pediatric neurosurgeon can be brought in to prepare for the implantation of a shunt shortly after birth.

As Sara Hannan recalled that conversation, Clewell explained the prenatal surgery but didn't push it on the couple. "Nothing against Dr. Clewell," she said, "but the doctors in Denver painted a really, really bleak picture for us. They said there are kids hospitalized with this condition, kids who are diapered when they are in their thirties. But they didn't push the surgery. They let us think about termination first. But we are of the Christian faith and we don't believe God makes mistakes. We couldn't consider termination."

The procedure was explained to the Hannans in detail, and team members told the couple that there is a small window in time, between the twentieth and thirtieth week of pregnancy, during which the procedure can be attempted—any earlier and the skull is too small to operate on, any later and it makes more sense to wait two more weeks, when the fetus can be delivered with a 95 percent chance of survival in the intensive care nursery. After telling the couple that the ventricles were taking up more than 70 percent of their baby's skull, the members of the fetal surgery team said, " 'Go home, decide, come back, and if you decide to terminate you can have it done here and go home and have a happy Christmas,' " Daniel Hannan said with a wry laugh. The couple opted for the uncertainty of the procedure over the certainty of abortion. The operation was scheduled for December 28.

Christmas of 1981 "was different from a lot of Christmases," Daniel Hannan said. "You ask a lot of questions that time of year: Why is this happening? Why is it happening to us? Why this time of year? But you make the best of it."

The couple returned to Denver on December 27, and the following morning Sara Hannan, "sedated but very much awake," lay on her back on an operating room table surrounded by "eighteen to twenty doctors at one time," as her husband describes it.

"They were all trying to look at this little eight-inch screen," he said. "It was comical really; the doctors didn't look at Sara, they were all watching that screen." Not only were the team members watching the screen, they were also watching a doll, which one of the physicians held in a position identical to that assumed by the fetus inside Sara Hannan. Thus Clewell and his associates were able to relate to a three-dimensional object as they inserted a needle through Hannan's abdomen and into the skull of the fetus. "They hold the baby from outside the mommy and press it in a certain position," Sara Hannan said. "You think mommies are supposed to be so careful with their tummies, and they are, but the doctors were really pushing hard, so hard they had to stop and shake their wrists every so often because they were getting sore. I was very much afraid. I guess I was in sort of a state of shock, but I was scared." The reason the staff members were pushing so hard was the need to keep the fetus from moving inside its liquid environment. Once it was positioned properly, and the procedure began, it was necessary to hold that position to insert the needle properly.

"The doctors told us they didn't know what would happen," Daniel Hannan said. "When they pushed that needle in it was like a sixteen penny box nail and it could kill the baby, it could go into his brain. We were anxious and nervous to see what would happen. We had prepared ourselves for the death of the child during the operation." Had the operation caused Nicholas's death, it would have been particularly hard on the parents, who had not only learned the sex through amniocentesis, but had already given the fetus a name and had been talking to him for weeks. While amniocentesis would not normally be part of a healthy twenty-six-year-old woman's pregnancy, Sara Hannan had undergone the procedure as one of many tests required for Nicholas's diagnosis and potential treatment.

An hour and a half after the procedure began, the doctors thought they had the shunt in place, and by the following day an ultrasound examination showed the ventricles greatly reduced as the fluid had drained into the amniotic sac. Then, twice a week for the next month, the couple was scheduled to make the three-hundred-mile round-trip drive to Denver for ultrasound examinations, but by about the twenty-sixth week it became apparent that Nicholas had pulled the shunt out, because the ventricles were enlarged even farther than they had been prior to the procedure. Thus a second attempt was made to insert a shunt, a procedure that took two and one-half hours, Sara Hannan recalled. "They about gave up the second time because they couldn't get him to hold still," she said. "They said they'd never seen such an active baby. After the first surgery he'd been much calmer, more peaceful, and he didn't kick as much. Then before the second surgery he'd been getting more active because he was in pain." Despite Nicholas's kicking, the surgeons managed to insert the second shunt in a better position than the first.

Things calmed down until February 26, 1982, when the Hannans returned to Denver for another of the biweekly ultrasounds. "I thought my amniotic fluid had begun leaking, and they told me they thought the ventricles were beginning to enlarge again," Sara Hannan said. "As I raised myself up from the table my water broke."

Three hours later, Nicholas Hannan was delivered by emergency cesarean section.

Premature delivery at thirty-two weeks did not end Nicholas's medical problems. They had, in fact, barely begun. The four-pound, three-ounce baby's lungs were compressed because he was suffering from a diaphragmatic hernia, a condition requiring surgical correction. In addition, he had a hole in one lung. By the time he was six months old he had undergone two operations on his diaphragm, an operation to implant another shunt to control his hydrocephalus and an operation on his lungs.

As of six months, however, all the correctable problems were corrected, according to Clewell. "He's developing," the surgeon said. "We're not sure he's going to be a completely normal child, but he's developing. You can't say much in the first months of life, but we have a follow-up program to at least age six to follow the development. In the long run, that's the most important part of our program"—to see if prenatal surgical intervention pays off in improved outcome for the babies involved.

In Nicholas Hannan's case, the point is debatable. His mother said that at age three he was "doing excellently as far as we're concerned" but "still has a long way to go."

"He has a great personality," Sara Hannan said. "He has a peaceful spirit."

But at age three Nicholas was described by developmental specialists as being on about a nine-month level. He couldn't talk, crawled on his back but not his front, and had not yet learned to sit up. By that time Nicholas had twice undergone surgery to correct his diaphragmatic hernia, had had a double hernia repaired, had had his shunt replaced and had required a gastrostomy—a surgically implanted feeding tube—because at a year and a half he weighed only fifteen pounds. "He had a problem with his stomach when he had all that diaphragm surgery," his mother explained. "He threw up all the time when he was a baby. They found out the top opening of his stomach was too large and they had to close it up. He had gotten to the point where he didn't want to drink or eat or anything."

Sara Hannan said she didn't know how much Nicholas's care had cost at that point, but she estimated it was in the hundreds of thousands of dollars. There had been no charge for the experimental fetal surgery, but the bill for Nicholas's initial surgery after birth and a month of neonatal care came to about $40,000, she said. After that, she said, the bills were paid by state and federal programs for handicapped children.

What of the future?

"We have a faith in God that we believe he's going to be healed, we know that the only way he's going to be all right is if he's healed," said Sara Hannan. "They wanted me to do the gastrostomy months before they did it. I wanted him to eat. He had so many surgeries before, I just didn't want to do any more. Now he's eating by mouth a little and he's progressing every day. I think in a couple of years he'll be able to eat all alone. I'm very pleased. I know that if he hadn't had that surgery before birth he'd be a lot worse. I know it's a success even if people look at him and don't think he's a success."

CHAPTER 6

Patients Before Birth

The cases of Michael Skinner and Nicholas Hannan provide a stark illustration of the risks and benefits of treating a patient as an experimental subject. The contrast between the success and what some might term failure is all the more tragic in these cases because of the age of the patients: They were fetuses, two potential children on the threshold of biologically independent life. These were not the usual subjects of human experimentation. They were not college students willing to take a minor risk to earn a few dollars. They were not terminally ill cancer patients, who, in most cases, had already lived a full life and might or might not have their lives extended a few more months or even years by an experimental therapy. And these were not fifty-five-year-olds with advanced heart disease, individuals so desperate to go on living they were willing to have an as yet unproven mechanical device implanted in their chests in the place of their own hearts.

Thus, these two cases also illustrate the two most difficult medical and ethical dilemmas facing physicians who would treat the fetus as a patient: If the treatment is not completely successful but the patient lives, the physician may have saved a horribly handicapped child for an entire lifetime of institutional existence, a child who might otherwise have been stillborn or might have died shortly after birth; and, by attempting the treatment in the first place, the physician is treating as a patient, and thus endowing with human value and rights, a fetus, an organism society has collectively—although not without much pain and dissension—agreed has no rights and may be killed upon the simple request of the woman carrying it.

Before considering these two issues, which lie at the core of any discussion of fetal therapy, it is necessary to understand where we stand today in terms of our ability to treat the fetus as patient. While some of the slightly more than one hundred surgical attempts worldwide to correct fetal defects have received a good deal of media attention, most human fetal treatments are still more conceptual than factual. The reality of the situation is that prenatal diagnosis has far outstripped medicine's ability to treat the myriad defects that can be detected prior to birth. Thus, in the vast majority of cases, ultrasound, amniocentesis and other diagnostic techniques are nothing more than early-warning systems, either providing worried parents with some degree of reassurance that their fetus is probably healthy and normal or, if that is not the case, giving them the choice of ending the pregnancy through abortion or preparing emotionally and medically for the birth of a sick or malformed newborn. Beyond that, however, there is little that can be done for the "defective" fetus. There are some conditions for which the mother's diet may be altered to protect the fetus from potential damage, such as diabetes, hypertension and PKU. And there have been a handful of cases worldwide of fetuses being treated in utero with vitamins or hormones to correct rare deficiencies or imbalances. There is, in fact, only one surgical fetal intervention that is now considered standard therapy, and that is intrauterine blood transfusion, first successfully completed in 1963.

Why attempt fetal therapy in the first place? Why not simply put our medical efforts and resources into treating those patients who are already born, and leave parents with their current choices: abort the "defective" fetus or attempt to correct its defect after birth? Because, said Dr. Michael Harrison, the medical issues in fetal therapy are similar to those in any other area of medicine. "Our problem in medicine at any age" is finding a condition too late to treat it. "Somebody finds out you have cancer of the lung and they say, 'God damn! I wish we were here six months ago so we could have fixed it. Now you're going to die.' Harrison is one of the co-directors of the fetal therapy program at the University of California at San Francisco. He is also co-author of *the* text on fetal therapy, *The Unborn Patient.* And it was Harrison and his team who, in what was the most dramatic fetal intervention thus far, partially removed a fetus from the uterus to correct a urinary tract blockage. Working through an incision in the abdomen and uterus, the surgeons temporarily "delivered" enough of the twenty-one-week fetus to make an incision and insert a catheter, or drainage tube, to drain the fetal urine into the amniotic fluid. Despite the technical success of the surgery, the infant died shortly after delivery at thirty-five weeks because its lungs had been so badly damaged by compression prior to the surgery. But it was the hope of saving such infants that drew Harrison into the field. To Harrison it seemed that "many kids could only be salvaged before birth. Clearly, from their physiology, that was the only time the babies could be salvaged."

As Harrison views it, fetal surgery has been made possible by several areas of medical endeavor and development, the first of which was having a group of surgeon-investigators who wanted to try it. The second was the development of an animal model of the disease process that needed correcting. Harrison and his group were inspired to try to correct lethal defects, and in the fetal lamb they had an animal model that various researchers had been developing and refining for more than two decades. Additionally, said Harrison, there was a third impetus coming from the clinical area, where the ability to diagnose prenatally almost a hundred conditions far outstripped the physician's ability to treat those conditions.

Starting in the late 1970s, Harrison and his group began approaching the possibility of fetal surgery as "a fraction of a fraction phenomenon," he said, sitting in his surgical scrub suit in his closet of an office. "You start out with a large number of problems that you find by accident. You narrow it down to a few that it would make any sense to treat before birth, so you've already excluded most of them, the ones that should be aborted, delivered early, delivered by C-section, have nothing done, transport the mom [to a high-risk center for delivery]. Then you have a small number that might deserve consideration for treatment before birth. First, there are the medical problems, and they're relatively large in number. Then there's a very small group of surgical problems: hydrocephalus, obstructed urinary tract—hydronephrosis, congenital diaphragmatic hernia. Now, the next important thing to point out is that of those problems, only a small fraction of fetuses who have those diagnoses made will require intervention, because all of those diseases come on a spectrum. The most severe on the spectrum won't make it no matter what, so if we get good enough at diagnosis, the answer would be to abort them. The most mild on the spectrum will probably get better no matter what we do." What is left, said Harrison, is a tiny group of fetuses, about one-third of the one in 500 fetuses affected by one of the three potentially surgically correctable conditions, who can be helped by surgical intervention in utero.

Two of the three conditions Harrison views as treatable; hydronephrosis and hydrocephalus are, as he puts it, "essentially drainage problems, so they're mechanically simple. Fluid's obstructed," he said, "and you need to make it flow. You can bypass the obstruction by having the fluid flow into the amniotic fluid." Most of the urinary tract problems can be corrected with a needle or catheter inserted through the mother's abdomen, eliminating the necessity to surgically open the abdomen and uterus and expose the fetus. But the thing that is most useful to families, said Harrison, is not necessarily having a procedure attempted but knowing that the problem exists. Then, he said, the woman can arrange to deliver her infant in a hospital that is prepared to operate on the infant at birth.

The most important thing, said Harrison, is not finding the fetus with a urinary tract blockage, but determining what the blockage means once it is found. And if that is to be done, someone must develop a test of fetal kidney function—simply determining the size of the kidney, or the area of damage, is not enough. What matters during the fetal period is how well the kidney is functioning and whether its output is blocked. If that can be accurately assessed, the need for surgery may become clearer. It may also then be easier to determine precisely which infants benefit from fetal intervention and which do not. The difference between fetal surgery to correct hydronephrosis and that to treat hydrocephalus is that the procedure for hydronephrosis is theoretically correcting the problem, while that for hydrocephalus is only, in theory, preventing further damage from occurring. And that is why Harrison's group has not attempted to treat children with hydrocephalus.

In the first place, Harrison said, although it is logical to assume that draining fluid prior to birth will prevent or reduce brain damage, no one has proven that. Additionally, not all hydrocephalus is caused by blocked fluid. "In some cases you have big ventricles and extra fluid because that goes with other intrinsic brain abnormalities." he said. "If you have a mechanical problem with obstruction to the flow of fluid and damage to the brain is secondary, it makes perfect sense" to relieve the pressure because "all the problem is is pressure squishing the brain. But what if you've got a collection of fluid that . . . is part of an intrinsic brain abnormality? Draining that fluid off is not going to help that kid one bit," said Harrison, who thinks researchers will eventually discover that hydrocephalus is a purely mechanical problem about 50 percent of the time.

But as Harrison and others in the field have asked on various occasions, while it is possible to create mechanically an animal model of hydrocephalus, and it is possible to determine if decompression reduces apparent brain damage, how can a researcher tell if the lamb, or, for that matter, the monkey, on whom he operated was or was not retarded? How can an animal model provide proof that relieving pressure on the fetal brain at a specific date saves the brain from damage? Dr. Frank Manning, professor and chairman of obstetrics and gynecology at the University of Manitoba in Canada, is one of those researchers who, like Harrison, has serious misgivings about prenatal surgical intervention in cases of hydrocephalus. Manning, who maintains an international fetal surgery registry and reports that there had been 72 bladder function problems and 32 cases of hydrocephalus reported by mid-1985, said the treatment of the bladder problems has been "quite encouraging: 45 percent of the fetuses treated have survived, most have been quite normal. That is encouraging viewed against the background that none of these children, or few of them, would have survived without the treatment. Hydrocephalus, on the other hand, is not a lethal disorder and you can't use simple survival to determine success," Manning said. "The real problem is whether or not you have normal development and whether or not you have improved the mental development of the child with therapy. We have seen five years of therapy," said Manning, whose own group does not attempt to correct hydrocephalus in the fetus. "We realize to our regret that normal survival is not the case: About one-third are normal and about two-thirds have minor to severe handicaps."

Does all of this effort make sense, in terms of the investment of manpower and resources, in a society that allows abortion? That, said UCSF's Harrison, is a "very difficult question. From the point of view of the things I actually deal with, like obstruction of the urinary tract and congenital diaphragmatic hernia [which he has repaired in animal fetuses but not in humans], there's no issue: The kids are going to die if you don't do it and they're potentially good kids. There are lots of kids walking around who had those lesions who were fixed early enough who are perfectly good kids, so there's no issue. And I don't think there's any issue in the big picture that it's worth it from the point of view of the input from society into that enterprise, because I think it's truly preventive medicine. If you look—and I'm very anxious to do it—at the cost of maintaining kids who are born with obstructed urinary tracts and kidney failures, well, that'll knock your eyeballs out, just with one or two of those kids. Renal failure in infancy," said Harrison, "is a terrible problem, and I think it would prove extremely cost-effective if you could prevent that.

"Now, you have to be extremely careful," he continued, "because what would be extremely cost-ineffectve would be if you take a bunch of kids who would die [without early intervention] and convert them to a bunch of kids with chronic renal failure. Now there is a tragedy. And that is the biggest danger of what we do, that we will fix kids halfway. That is a potential tragedy of the first order. And if you think it's a tragedy with the urinary tract, which it is, think of how awful it is for hydrocephalus—which is another reason we're going to go slow with that enterprise, because the stakes are so much higher. You take a kid who would die at birth, who had a horrible malformation, and you halfway fix him to a kid who's retarded and malformed and just awful—Jeeees! That would prove terribly cost-ineffective and morally reprehensible."

But what does the ability to treat fetuses as patients do to the abortion debate? Quite simply, Harrison responded, it turns the debate around. Fetal therapy, he said, is not a public health issue: "The diseases are all very rare. But as an ethical and philosophical issue, it has immense impact, even if you can only fix one in a million as opposed to fixing none in a million. And the reason it turns it around is this: Prenatal diagnosis has always been tainted by the end product—because, hell, I mean the only thing you were doing that stuff for, the tremendous effort in prenatal diagnosis, was to bump off the kid. And that's basically what it was. Now if you have even a few of those problems that you can potentially fix, it changes the whole emphasis. Now you can say we're screening one thousand kids to find the one who's fixable, instead of screening one thousand kids to kill everybody that isn't like us."

Unfortunately, the abortion debate and the philosophical questions raised about fetal surgery are far more complicated than Harrison's rationale would suggest. Consider, once again, the examples of Nicholas Hannan and Michael Skinner. As fetuses at the time they were surgically treated, not only would they not normally be considered "patients," they would normally not even be considered "persons" in the eyes of the law. They lay, and such patients continue to lie, in a truly schizophrenic social, legal and medical no-man's-land. On one hand, in order to protect the "rights" of fetuses and even human embryos, the National Institutes of Health has issued strict guidelines severely limiting research and experimentation involving embryos and fetuses, including those that are severely deformed and/or quite clearly will not survive gestation. On the other hand, society legally sanctions abortion—the killing of embryos and fetuses—for whatever reason the pregnant woman deems appropriate. Thus, we forbid researchers to conduct experiments upon fetuses that are about to be, or have just been, aborted, despite the fact that those experiments could provide invaluable knowledge about fetal physiology, treatment and disease, and yet we allow a fetus to be aborted simply because it is female and its parents want a boy, or its mother is up for a promotion in her job and isn't ready to take a pregnancy leave.

New York University philosophy professor William Ruddick doesn't see any difficulty in saving a fetus on one floor of a hospital while aborting a fetus on another. "I don't think there is any inconsistency in struggling to save something others do not want, and vice versa," he said. As Ruddick views it, "the issue as it is being debated is: If a fetus becomes a patient, doesn't that mean the fetus is a person and doesn't that show that abortion is wrong? . . . This is totally wrong," he said. "You can call a sick pet a patient. What's more, this argument doesn't take into account the reality: Being a patient means being stripped of the sort of things we associate with being a person," such as autonomy, independence, privacy and dignity. "If anything, being a patient counts against retaining status as a person. Whether someone has status as a person is usually a matter of legal or religious decision.

"These discussions are at the level of polemic," Ruddick said. "The people have already reached moral opinions and adopted a terminology appropriate to it. If you believe for metaphysical reasons that the fetus is a spiritual equal, you will talk about mother and child from day one. If you don't hold that view and want to ensure that women are not subject to certain moral or legal restrictions, then you will hold off talking about a 'child' until the birth.

"The problem about the options that medicine creates is that once they are developed they create not only options but obligations, and if that doesn't happen, the increasing refinements lead to more and more use where" the potential benefit is questionable at best. And, Ruddick added, "What makes the fetal thing more complicated is all this political and metaphysical debate

118

about personhood. The serious debate, I think, is about women: whether motherhood is a natural and obligatory situation in women."

What Ruddick is referring to is a question that concerns many other ethicists, philosophers and legal scholars: If we have the ability to provide unquestionably beneficial fetal therapy, are we obligated to provide it? If we are, how do we balance the conflicting rights of the two patients in each case, the mother and the fetus?

John Robertson, a law professor at the University of Texas at Austin and a specialist in the rights of the handicapped, notes that conflict arises not in a case where a woman does want to abort a defective fetus, but rather, where she knows she is carrying a defective fetus, wants to continue with the pregnancy, *and* there is a viable treatment available for the defect. Clearly, he said, such treatment is in the interest of most such women, who would be happy to have the fetal defect treated. The conflict arises, said Robertson, only if a woman "refuses the treatment that was established as helpful to her child-to-be. At that point we have a conflict with the mother's wishes and the interests of the future child."

Robertson makes an important point here, for he is not talking about conflicting rights of woman and fetus. Other than those taking an uncompromising antiabortion position, no one is really raising the issue of "fetal rights" in this discussion because society has determined that if the mother does not want to carry her fetus to term, it has no rights (other than protection from experimentation) prior to the point of viability. There is, for instance, no question here of determining via proxy what the "wishes" of the fetus might be. But what Robertson is talking about are the conflicting rights of mother and child, for the given in the discussion is that the woman *wants* the fetus she is carrying and will continue to carry it. "We're not really talking about the

119

fetus's right to have treatment," Robertson points out, "we are really talking about the right of the child who is going to be born to be born healthy. . . . We are talking about the future child. The child that the mother has decided to have. If there were a conflict between the child she decided to have and what she wants done, it seems to me that ethically and legally the interests of the child should take priority. She has an obligation to that child once she chooses to have that child."

On the other hand, NYU's Ruddick views the dilemma from the viewpoint of the mother, stating that "women should have the liberty to define the obligations they are willing to undertake. The fact that they started out on a project that has gone seriously bad doesn't commit them to continuing that project come what may. . . . It should be up to the woman to redefine the project. It is important to note, obviously, that once past a certain point, some projects must be completed for legal reasons.

"But I think discussing the 'best interests of the child' is importing into these decisions notions of the law that were developed with much older and more developed human beings in mind. It seems to me fairly easy to say in children of four or five, 'What is in the best interests of the child?' But in these cases, what's in the best interest is still hard to define.

"I don't see how there is enough known by anybody to make these [conflict of interest] decisions," Ruddick continued. "It is hard enough to separate off in early infancy, let alone earlier, the parental interests, the child's interests, and then ask: Whose interests are going to rule? Generally we believe that the interests of an infant and its parents are so bound up together that you can't define them independently. Certainly it can't be in our interests as parents to let our children suffer. But it is too simple to set this up as a dilemma between parental interests and child's interests. In the case of a pregnant woman with a fetus diagnosed as seriously imperiled, there is only one set of interests and that is not because the fetus counts as nothing. It is rather that the interests of a pregnant woman wanting to have a child prevail."

Bioethicist John C. Fletcher is even more troubled than Ruddick, if that is possible, by the possibility that society might adapt Robertson's view of conflicting maternal-fetal rights. "We have to take a stand now because our society is going through changes, and these techniques are creating stars in people's eyes. The mother's interests come first whenever you have to go through her body to treat the fetus, with one exception: when the condition is life-threatening to both mother and fetus, for example in placenta previa, where the placenta blocks the opening of the [uterus]—if you don't intervene there you would have a dead baby and a dead mother. But we should not violate or coerce women against their will," Fletcher said. "Then we would have a health police state to monitor pregnancies. Women should not be exempt from the consent form. Pregnancy is not a jail sentence," the noted bioethicist said. "I am opposed to coercive fetal therapy or surgery."

IV.
BORN AT RISK

CHAPTER 7

A Very Wanted Child

He is a physicist in his early forties. She is a theoretical mathematician and college professor. That they had been married for fifteen years prior to her becoming pregnant had nothing to do with fertility, but rather, bespoke a dedication to career and being "ready" for parenthood. "This was a very planned-for, wanted child," the father said, explaining that he and his wife tried to anticipate everything about the birth of their first child. For example, they had arranged, with some difficulty, to take leaves from work at the same time, so that they could be home for at least a month. Then, too, said the father, "We'd tried to think of the various things that could go wrong, and this wasn't the type of thing that entered our minds."

It's not that the couple hadn't considered the possibility of health problems, but, as the thirty-five-year-old woman explained, she and her husband had worried about her health, never considering that their baby might have a problem. There had been one previous, unplanned pregnancy, in 1977. But because the woman had been taking heavy medication for a thyroid condition, her physicians had advised her to abort. There was a chance, the doctors said, that the medication might have damaged the fetus. By 1983, however, the thyroid condition had been brought under control, and its only remaining manifestation was moderate hypertension. "Before we became pregnant my blood pressure was a little on the high side—130 or 140 over 90—which my obstetricians felt, if it were well controlled and monitored, I should be able to risk this. And I became pregnant in May."

"The first two trimesters were very smooth," the father recalled. "We did have an amnio done at the sixteenth week, and it showed a healthy, growing baby girl fetus." Throughout her pregnancy, the woman was monitored carefully by a group of obstetricians specializing in high-risk pregnancies and by a hypertension specialist. In early October, during a weekly examination, a dangerously high blood-pressure reading of 220 over 120 was recorded. One of the doctors wanted to put her in the hospital right away, the mother said. "Because I had been fighting this hypertension for a number of years," she said, "and I had been monitored by an expert in hypertension in pregnancy, I thought he was overreacting. I yelled at him—which showed that I was in trouble!" But another expert in hypertension, asked for a second opinion, also insisted on hospitalizing her, and she was admitted for about four days of testing and observation. That led doctors to start her on minimal doses of a drug to control the hypertension.

"I had resisted going on any medication," she said, "because of the risk to the fetus. I felt that if I could have bed rest until she was big enough to be delivered. . . . All through the pregnancy I'd noticed that my psychological frame of mind was almost the best in my life," the mother said. "I had been plagued throughout my life by being negative, and being pessimistic, and harking back on my past and going into rages. . . . But throughout the pregnancy I was extremely mellow, I felt more happy, more peaceful. Initially I had doubts about whether I'd be a good mother and how this would change our life—I feel guilty about that—but into the second trimester I was very upbeat, very confident—it was almost a euphoria. I noticed toward the end, however, that my old irritability was coming back." At least one physician theorized the mood change was being caused by increasingly high blood pressure.

On Friday, November 9, the mother was examined by a prominent specialist in high-risk pregnancy and fetal development. He was somewhat reassured by what he found, the mother recalled. But she said: "One thing that stuck in my mind, that's plagued me ever since, was he took my hand and he said—I was in my twenty-eighth week—'If the baby is born now, the neonatologist will perhaps give you an optimistic view that the baby has an eighty-percent chance of survival. But I will tell you it has a fifty-percent chance of survival, and of those fifty percent, half of those will have something seriously wrong with them.' So he said, in that very effusive Italian way that he has, 'So, my darling, if you can hold on for three more weeks, the baby at thirty-two weeks then definitely has a close to eighty-percent chance of survival.' He said, in essence, these are the three most important weeks of your pregnancy. And to such a large extent I feel like I failed so much, I wasn't able to get through the three most important weeks of my pregnancy, and it just eats at me so much." The woman wept.

"You can't control . . . ," her husband tried to console her.

"I know, intellectually I know that," she said, "but the fact that he said that, and the fact that it happened and I couldn't hold on, has been the most haunting thing. . . ."

During the weekend, the woman began to have difficulty urinating, and between Saturday and Monday she gained eleven pounds. Even more alarming was a finding of protein in her urine, a sign, along with the weight gain, that the woman was developing severe preeclampsia, potentially life-threatening hypertension in pregnancy. She was immediately admitted to the hospital again.

Things went well her first day there, November 12. Her blood pressure came down a bit, and she lost some weight. But the following day is one neither parent will ever forget. About 7:45 A.M., just before leaving for work, the father telephoned the nurses' station. "The nurse told me a resident had just finished a fairly complete physical and it looked like things were coming along," the father said. "Then I went to work, and I expected [my wife] to call me when she woke up. I didn't really worry, but there was a normal break in my work around ten o'clock, a little after ten, so I called her room and I didn't get any answer," he said. "So that worried me, but I thought she might be in the bathroom. I waited five minutes and I called back, and I still didn't get any answer. So I called the nurses' station, and the nurse said, 'Oh yes, we were thinking about calling you. . . . Your wife's been transferred down to the delivery room. This doesn't necessarily mean she's going to have to be delivered, but we felt that under the circumstances it should be done.' "

The father immediately took a cab to the hospital. "I ran into the delivery area," he said. "First thing, I was stopped by a nurse who said I had to put on a gown just to be in a delivery area. They said, 'Yes, your wife is down here, she's in a room being monitored.' " As he was changing into a light green hospital gown, a specialist whom his wife had consulted a few days earlier approached the father. "He said, 'We're going to have to deliver your wife. It's a matter of her life. We don't have any choice. I'm sorry.' "

The baby would be delivered, the father was told, by the senior partner in the group that had been caring for the mother.

The father entered his wife's labor room. "She had a continuous blood-pressure monitor attached to her arm," he said. "They were pumping her full of [drugs] to get it down, and the nurse told me that before they brought her down it was reading 230 over 125, and it was reading 190 over 115 when I walked into the room, and I was just stunned by the whole thing. I had expected something like another three-day stay and maybe they'd change the medication she was getting," the father said. "I had foreseen the possibility they might want to hospitalize her for the duration, I had come to terms with that. . . ." His voice trailed off.

The mother, too, was scared by the speed with which her pregnancy was ending. "I knew that if they gave me gas it would lessen her [the baby's] chances because she would get a knockout dose, too," the mother said. "I was determined to give her every chance I could, so I asked if it was possible to give me an epidural [spinal anesthesia], and they said yes, they could give me an epidural but they wanted to do it fast."

While his wife was wheeled into the delivery room and prepared for an emergency cesarean section, her husband and the obstetrician stood together at a stainless-steel sink as the physician scrubbed his hands and arms to the elbows. "I still was in shock and not understanding what had happened," the father recalled. "I just stood there as he scrubbed—it takes a lot longer for a real doctor to scrub than in the movies. I asked him what had happened, and he said she had gone into acute preeclampsia and that it was life-threatening, her blood pressure was in what he said was 'stroke territory,' that a stroke could occur at any instant really, and that the only known treatment for this condition was to end the pregnancy, no matter what.

"My wife has always had a problem healing with scars," the father continued, "and I knew from my reading that it was quite common in emergency C-sections to do a vertical cut, which wouldn't heal as readily. I said, 'I know this is true, and I'm not a doctor, but do you think it would be possible to do a transverse cut?' He thought about it for several minutes and then said, 'Yes,

we can try that, I don't think it will make much difference.' "
The father sighed, and there were tears in his eyes. "As it turned
out, I have since felt a little guilty about that conversation. . . ."

"No," his wife interrupted, quietly but firmly, "I also asked
for it."

The delivery proved to be difficult. The surgery was begun so
soon after the anesthetic was administered that the mother felt
the cutting and had to be given more medication. The father
kept popping up from his seat by his wife's head, looking over
the surgical drape that was meant to screen the incision from his
view. "I kept saying, 'It's okay, it's okay,' but what I was seeing
wasn't okay," he said. "Both the resident and obstetrician were
really tugging inside of her, and every so often I'd see this little
blue arm coming out the opening and they'd say, 'No, not the
arm.' What had happened was that at this unfortunate instant the
baby was in a transverse position and they couldn't get either the
butt or the head. The resident became very agitated, not in his
movement but in his facial expressions, and saying to anybody
around him, 'We've got to get her out quick.' "

It was another five minutes before the obstetrician finally
managed to grasp the baby's head and tug her free of the uterus.
"She was the color of your shirt"—blue—said the father, "and
absolutely lifeless. I remember saying to myself, 'The baby's
dead.' At the same time I was saying to my wife, 'It'll be all
right, it's just about over.' I sat down and saw the neonatologist
rushing over to the baby. It couldn't have been more than a minute later we heard two small little cries. It was another shock to
me. I just thought the baby was dead, that was it. But the cries
were definitely a baby's cries. They'd resuscitated her on the first
try. I said, 'It's all right, the baby's alive.' "

So on November 13, 1984, the baby girl for whom her parents had hoped and planned entered the world, approximately
ten weeks early, weighing two pounds, nine ounces. And as her

mother was being cleaned up and prepared for admission to the adult intensive care unit, the doll-sized infant was rushed to the neonatal intensive care unit.

"I don't remember too much of the day," the father said, holding his wife's hand. "I remember going into the nursery and seeing them put the baby on oxygen. Then I went to see my wife."

The neonatal intensive care unit was not at all what he expected. "The first thing I saw was a long bench, where they do the tests. . . . I thought, 'Gee, it's like a chemistry lab bench.' "

As the mother was wheeled through the nursery on her way to the adult ICU, she had her first glimpse of the baby. "I remember thinking how long she was," the mother recalled, "and how boiled lobster red she was."

The father said that the next several days were a blur, filled as they were with fears for his wife's life and forty-mile round trips between the couple's suburban home and the downtown hospital. "In the first couple days when I went home, I rarely thought about the baby," he said. "My thoughts were on my wife. . . . The baby seemed to be alive and they were doing what they could, but it really wasn't in my thoughts, just my wife, because she did look so strange. I knew that wasn't right. I didn't need to have any blood types done or anything. She looked sick. And I had read that sometimes even ending the pregnancy does not stop the eclampsia, and that's what I was really scared about. I was really scared about strokes. 'Cause I had a history professor in college who had a number of strokes. The third one finally killed him, and the first two paralyzed him in various ways. One of the most brilliant men I've ever met. But he had his first stroke when he was sixty-something, and to think of my wife like that was . . ." Again his voice trailed off.

The couple recalled that the neonatologist initially caring for their baby had a very subdued demeanor. "He would come in, no smiles, and just be very—he wasn't cold, he was clinical, businesslike," the mother said. "He'd give me readouts, blood gases, which I didn't understand at the time. He'd say she's very sick. He'd say she needs lots of support, but she's stable. And I would just thank him. I didn't have anything else to ask him. I wanted to ask him questions, but I just didn't know anything to ask."

Said the father: "I guess the only thing I asked him at the time was, 'Do you think she was without oxygen long enough to sustain brain damage?' And he said he couldn't be sure, but he felt that the odds were pretty strong against it because, one, apparently it takes a longer time to sustain brain damage with an infant than with an adult, and, secondly, the time between when she was detached from the placenta to when she was resuscitated was at most two to three minutes, so he felt that was not a problem. He felt her basic problem was the shock of how she was delivered, and he said very early that he felt her lungs were very immature."

By Sunday, five days after the baby was born, things were looking up. The neonatologist who had resuscitated the baby came to visit the mother, who recalled: "She was actually smiling, it was the first time we'd seen any of them smile. Our baby was doing beautifully, they had her oxygen down to forty-five percent, her blood gases were good. . . . So I was ecstatic. That evening our friends came and brought a little premie outfit as a gift," she said. "I was so worried about my husband at that point, because of the double strain on him worrying about me and the baby, that I wanted him to have a break. And their gift to me was to take him out to dinner. . . . In the interim though, while they were out to dinner, the resident came in and I was running a temperature. And they decided to open up a couple of stitches and, sure enough, I was infected. So in the two hours my husband was out to dinner they cleaned me out, and I was in agony. I thought I was screaming. . . . I was happy my husband wasn't there, because I didn't want this on top of everything else. . . . It was awful."

The mother was placed in isolation because of her infection, unable to visit her baby—who also had a troubled night. "I felt like I was sending these strong psychic waves down to the baby to hang on," she said. "But it was ironic: Sunday morning when I was doing well and feeling on top of the world, the baby was doing well; Sunday night when I went down, she went down. It's so incredible that she was going down when I was going down."

"But still," the father said, "they were saying she'd be so much better if they could get her off the respirator, but the neonatologist on that rotation was still saying that he felt that the long-range prognosis was positive. I got fixated on all the numbers. Numbers are my business. I went over how accurate are these? Is the last significant digit really a significant digit? It usually turned out the answer was no. I got fixated on that, but the baby was responsive. That seemed so wonderful to me. You scratched its feet, and it would kick its feet. It would grab your finger, not like a real infant, but it would definitely curl its fingers around the finger. . . . Finally my wife got out of isolation," he said. "When she came down and talked to her, she opened her eyes for the first time." Before, their daughter's lids had only been seen fluttering.

The baby also had begun to respond to voices, a nurse told them. "When my wife started talking to her and touching her, her absorption of oxygen went up," the father said. "It turned out later that whenever either one of us spoke to her and touched her at the same time we could see her respond by her blood oxygen going up."

The Tuesday before Thanksgiving, November 20, when the baby was one week old, her mother was discharged from the hospital. While at least the couple was reunited, now both the father and the mother, who was not up to traveling back and forth, needed to commute to see their baby. At first, except for Thanksgiving Day—when they followed the neonatologist's advice to take a breather—the father would go to the hospital at least once a day. The couple remained optimistic, "although," the father said, "we'd already been told by the neonatologist that the longer she was on oxygen, the worse it was." He said: "The next week I think I went to work one or two days. It was very difficult for my wife to get around, so I went every day to the NICU [neonatal intensive care unit] and we'd call every couple of hours to get reports."

On November 29, the father went to work and his wife traveled to the city herself around noon for an appointment with a hypertension specialist and a visit to the nursery. About 3:45, recalled the father, "the doctor called me at work, and . . . he said, he started out with, 'I'm sorry. It's very bad. I don't think she's going to make it today. You'd better come down here immediately.' I think I called my father, who also works downtown, and said, 'The baby's dying. Could you come down and be with us.' I rushed down, and the baby had developed several pneumothoraxes [air pockets in the chest cavity that can cause a lung to collapse], and the blood gases had gone to hell and they had put a tube in her chest to try to take out the air that had gotten into the chest from the pneumothorax. But they didn't expect her to survive. The social worker was there, and I met the minister for the first time. My father arrived and we—"

His wife continued: "I called my psychiatrist, who's a good friend, and said, 'Please come, my baby's dying.' So we all congregated in the family room, and we thought that at any moment she would expire. But she pulled through."

"The neonatologist had given us no hope," the father said. "November 29 was going to be it. But around seven, eight o'clock, she stabilized—at a higher level of support, but she was stabilized. . . . But when we went home I remember asking

134

them, 'Is it possible that if the baby dies during the night you can wait to call us in the morning?' "

The mother said that she explained, " 'We have to get some sleep, and there's nothing we can do.' "

The father continued: "And they said, 'Well, I don't know what the legal standing is but I think we can do that.'

"The next morning when we called in she'd had a good night. They'd been able to cut down on the oxygen some—she was down to sixty-five to seventy percent—and she was doing better. So we decided to come in and see her late Friday."

On Friday, November 30, when the couple made their daily visit late in the afternoon, they learned that their baby had suffered another pneumothorax. "They didn't think it was as serious as the first one, but it was serious," the father said. "But she pulled through that one."

The following Monday promised to be a particularly difficult day for the family. Because of the extraordinary psychological and physical strains on neonatologists, most nurseries establish staffing patterns in which each of the senior neonatologists is on "clinical rotation" for a month at a time and attends to administration or research for the next month. While this makes life a bit easier for the doctors, it means that each month parents must establish a relationship with another physician. "They said that Monday [December 3], the head neonatologist would come on rotation," said the father. "We hadn't met him, but we had an idea about him. The social worker had already warned us that he's very direct. I said, 'Good!' "

"I liked the other doctor [the one who had been caring for the baby during November]," said the mother, "but he was a little unwilling to say anything. He was too wishy-washy. He'd say could, could not, could, could not. I needed some bluntness at that point. . . ."

While the parents were still hopeful that their baby would ulti-

135

mately recover, the daily crisis-to-crisis nature of her course had pushed them to the point of some very tentative discussions with the first neonatologist about how long the doctors could keep trying. The father said he asked, " 'How long can she stay on the system and how much discomfort is she in?' " And he recalled the doctor saying, " 'We don't want the baby to suffer. This isn't the sort of place where we make the babies suffer. But we're trying to give her all the support we can.' And he explained that some of the support was hurting her, the excessive amounts of oxygen, and she had these young lungs without the surfactant [naturally produced chemical] to keep the air bags open. . . ."

After the first pneumothorax, said the father, the neonatologist had told the parents the baby had a secondary condition, bronchopulmonary dysplasia, that the doctors thought was caused by the respirator. "He said that, in addition, there might be a virus or fungus infection. They'd done some tests for fungus, but that's hard to do. And they'd done some tests for virus, but they're hard to do and are of questionable worth because even if they found a virus infection, there wasn't anything they could do about it. So he said he didn't really know what was wrong. Her heart was strong and steady, beating a steady one hundred fifty beats a minute, it hardly ever changed," the father said. "The IVs [intravenous lines] kept slipping out, and I remember they had called me at home like Tuesday, November 27, and said we just need your permission to perform a small operation to surgically implant the IV. . . . I said, sure, go ahead, if that's all you're calling me for. . . . She was very active, almost too active. They were even thinking of sedating her."

Indeed, on the thirtieth, after the second major crisis, the baby was given Pavulon, a paralyzing agent, to keep her from fighting against the respirator tube and other monitor leads and lines that were draped across her tiny body. "That was very discouraging to us because she could no longer respond, all her muscles were paralyzed, although she'd still respond with the absorption of the oxygen."

Monday, December 3, the father took the afternoon off from work, and he and his wife went to the nursery to meet with the hospital's director of neonatology. "He was different from what I pictured from the descriptions. He wasn't as overwhelmingly physically imposing as the descriptions had made you think," the father said. "This was also the first time we'd ever talked to a doctor in a doctor's office. He took us back into his office and sat us down and said we had a very sick baby and he saw only three possible courses:

"One was to go on as they were doing, and it was possible the baby would come out of it because it was a very strong baby in recovering but it kept having these crises and after each crisis it was worse. The past night at two A.M. she had had a very bad pneumothorax on the other side. He said, 'I really do not see a favorable prognosis as likely if we keep going the way we are.'

"He said a second possibility would be 'to take her off the respirator and let nature take its course. Of course, I could not take her off oxygen because that would be cruel, and I would certainly give her morphine to make sure she would not be in any pain, and I would tell you the odds are very great that she could not live for more than a couple of hours off the respirator.' He said, 'I am willing to discuss that at this time if you want to.'

" 'The third possibility,' " the father remembers being told, " 'is to give her some steroids. This is, at present, experimental. We are actually running an experiment now in the hospital, and your baby would not be eligible for the experiment because we have a cutoff point of being on the respirator thirty days. And anyway I don't feel your baby would be a candidate, because we want to definitely give her the steroids and while the test is going on it's a double-blind test where we wouldn't know whether the baby is getting the steroids or not. We'd see how she's responding to it in three or four days.'

"Then I asked him about damage to the baby's eyes and damage to the baby's brain," the father said. "He said that at this point he saw no evidence that there'd be significant damage. . . . He said, 'We'll reassess everything and why don't we plan to have a long talk on Friday afternoon.' "

"We opted for number three," the father said. "We said, as long as there's a chance, let's try it. Yes, it was experimental, yes, they only had anecdotal information, but let's try it. They gave her a shot, and within an hour after the shot, the baby's blood oxygen just shot up."

"We thought that this was the miracle we needed," the mother said. By Tuesday morning the baby's blood-oxygen reading was in the 60s, and the physicians were able to slightly reduce the percentage of pure oxygen the respirator delivered. The director said, " 'If it gets into the 70s, we'll cut back the oxygen more.' I was there at the time, just waiting for the next blood gas, and it came back at 71 and the nurses and I were so elated. But do you know that five minutes later, just about four in the afternoon . . . she blew another pneumothorax, a big one," said the mother, her voice drowning in tears.

"And the blood oxygen dropped lower than it ever had and she had great trouble coming back up at all," her husband continued. "The most she got back to was the 40s. . . ."

"I went in by myself December the fifth," the mother said, "and I said to the neonatologist, 'I know that you had planned to cut the cortisone and just give her a four-day regimen, give her two days of full shots and then two days of half-strength shots, but I'm willing to do anything, even if it kills her. This is experimental. If at the end of the four days you feel she has any kind of a chance, will you start the treatment over? Because I feel that the experiment has been muddied, because she was doing so well

138

and then she blew a pneumothorax.' I will never know, if the luck had been with her, and she hadn't blown the pneumothorax, maybe the cortisone would have kept her at that 70 level. I can't tell now. And he said, 'Sure. I'm relieved. I thought you were going to ask me to try something else, and I don't have anything in my bag of tricks to give you.' That was Wednesday.''

"She was not doing well, and the really bad thing was they got another set of X-rays of her lungs and I got to see them," the father said. "And even for a totally nonmedical person the lungs didn't look like any shape lungs I'd ever seen before. One lung was pear shape, or maybe you'd call it butternut squash shape, with a long neck and a big bulge at the bottom, a bulge so big that it went over into the other side of the chest. Then the lung on the other side was like a real acute triangle. It really came to a point. . . . Also, we felt very much that day, December 6, at least I felt, that the attitude of the doctors had changed. In a way they all, especially the nurses, had been really upbeat and felt she was such a fighter . . . in spite of all the medical numbers coming back."

Said the mother, "In fact, nurses became very attached to her because she was such a fighter. They told me they'd never seen a baby fight so hard."

"But," the father continued, "I think all the nurses, many more than were assigned to her, came over and looked at the X-rays. . . . To them I guess it was a thing of saying, 'Well, we can't ignore the objective medical findings anymore. This baby's losing it, in spite of her fighting.' So we went in to talk to the director."

"I'd gone in in the morning myself," the mother said. "I always, before I scrubbed, looked in, and the doctor and several nurses and the resident were all hovered around her, and so I knew something was up. And the director looked up and we locked eyes, for about a full minute, and I could tell by his eyes

139

that something was terribly wrong and my heart knew that it was over." She began crying softly. "I didn't want to verbalize it, but I knew by the way that he looked at me through the glass, that we looked at each other and locked eyes, I knew that it was over. I scrubbed anyway, and before I got in he came out and said, 'Let's go to my office.' He said essentially that before I came in the morning her heart had failed and they'd had a hard time getting her back up the first time and it failed again. And he said, 'I don't know if we can get it back up again. I'm sorry, but I think this is it. Maybe you'd better call your husband.'"

Her husband, too, was crying at this point in their narration. "And so she called me at work and said that our daughter had died, and that her heart had given out. . . ."

"Her strong heart . . . ," her mother said, barely audible.

". . . Her strong heart," echoed her husband. "I got down to the NICU—"

"But before he got down," his wife interrupted, her tears changing to the laughter that can appear so incongruously in the midst of grief, "I expected that she was dead, but then the doctor came out after I called my husband, and he leaned against the wall and said, 'I don't believe it, but she's pulled out of this one. The roller coaster starts again.' And I just wept openly, and I said, 'I can't take this, I just can't take this.' At the same time I was thanking God or whoever is up there. I said, 'She's been resurrected. I can't believe it,' and he said, 'Neither can I. I don't know what's keeping this baby alive.' Then my husband arrived and we went into the director's office, and we essentially asked, what we wanted was, we don't want a brilliant child, we just want a healthy, happy child. . . ."

"We just want a child that . . . ," began the father, who then continued, in perfect, spontaneous unison with his wife, ". . . eventually will be able to take care of itself."

"Not even healthy at first," said the father, alone. "We realized that would be unlikely—but eventually could make its own way in the world. . . . He [the director] left the room for a minute and then came back. He said her heart was still not functioning right and the resident was hovering over her and the blood-oxygen levels were still very low. And I said, 'What's your prognosis right now?' And he said, 'I don't believe the baby can live another day, no matter what we do.'

"I said, 'How about more steroids?' And he said, 'No. We've tried it enough. There really hasn't been anything positive from the steroids.' I said, 'This is all experimental. She did improve, she did go up for the day. Let's say you were writing this up for a paper you were preparing to publish on the effects of steroids,' and he's very bright, he saw where I was heading, and he interrupted and he said, 'I would have to call this attempt a failure.' "

Continued the father, "I said, 'Well, what if you could wave a magic wand right now and the baby would get better but the damage she sustained wouldn't change? She'd be as damaged as she is right now. What sort of existence do you see for her?'

"And he said, 'Well, she's going to, her lungs are going to be very badly damaged for a long time. She's going to need considerable support here, and when you go home you're going to need oxygen and she's going to need considerable support, massive operations. The heart is also probably damaged now, probably due to oxygen deprivation.' The first thing he said was the motor centers, which I had never thought about, were probably damaged. Of course the brain controls the motor centers, but I had only thought about intellectual ability. He said, 'She probably won't be able to move around very well.' I said, 'What about retardation?' And he said, 'Yes . . . I would say significant retardation.' "

The doctor reminded the parents it was impossible to test the baby because she was on Pavulon. "I said, 'You really don't expect her to live past Friday'—this was Thursday—'do you?' And he said, 'Well, anything can happen. The baby's a fighter, but I would really be surprised if she could last into the weekend.' He said, 'Right now I feel there's a third heart failure about to happen.' Then I think he brought it up to take her off the respirator. I might have brought it up earlier in talking about the possibilities."

About a week earlier the husband and wife had talked together about the possibility of having their daughter removed from the respirator at some point. "We just basically said as long as she had a chance for a quasi-normal life without pain, we didn't even want to consider taking her off," said the father. The bottom line, he said, was that she live a life free of pain, and he and his wife were "very much aware that we were elderly [first-time parents] and I couldn't see her being institutionalized at thirty and being kept next to a vegetable and existing. . . . Self-sufficiency is what we wanted. But if you could have promised us a full, pain-free life—but she might have to be institutionalized at some point—I don't know what we'd have. . . ."

His wife picked up the story. "The neonatologist said, 'I don't want you to worry about the [Baby Doe] hotline. In this case I would take care of it completely. I don't think there would be any questions.' "

"I said, 'Yeah, I don't need Jesse Helms in my life,' " the father said bitterly. "Maybe my wife said, 'Do you have to convene an ethics committee?' " the father recalled. "And the director said, 'Well, you know, this hospital doesn't have an ethics committee. . . . I could get everything set up in twenty minutes.' I said, 'We were talking about making a decision Friday, but we could make it today.' By this time we were pretty mixed up and everything. He said, 'I don't want to pressure you at all into anything. I have to go on rounds. You can either make up your mind sometime today, or sometime tomorrow, or not at all.'

"He left us alone with the social worker," said the father, "and we sort of said, 'Should we wait till tomorrow?' . . . We talked to the social worker and she said, 'What are you going to do tonight if you don't make a decision?' And we said to each other that it just didn't seem to make any sense putting off a decision, and it seemed to us that the only two possibilities were wait for nature to take its course and have what the doctors considered an almost inevitable third heart attack that they wouldn't be able to bring her back from, or" —he sighed—"to take her off the respirator and be able to hold her for the first time even if it would be the last time." He continued: "In a way, it wasn't a difficult decision to say, 'Take her off the respirator.' We had no feeling that we were killing her. There was a question of now or an hour later— or which way we could comfort her and ourselves the most. That was the only question. The doctor said he had exhausted everything he could do. As far as he could see the baby was dying and dying rapidly. He said there was no way to stop the deterioration that he knew of.

"When he came back in he said, 'Fine.' He didn't argue with us at all about our decision . . . ," the father continued. "We said again that we didn't want her to be in any pain, and he said, 'I'll be sure of that. I'm going to give her a shot of morphine.' " The father continued: "They set up a screen around the table and we went in. She had most of the tubes out of her. They still had the chest tubes for the pneumothorax in her, but they were no longer connected to the suction pump. For the first time we could see her face completely, unencumbered by the braces that held the respirator tube. And we held her. During the entire time we held her, the total time was about an hour, an hour and a half. Her heart was still beating, she was still breathing. Then she gasped, and they gave her some more morphine. Her heart rate dropped down to about 16. They'd warned us that she might live for several hours. I called my father and said her heart's still beating but down. Then I bumped into the director, and I said, 'Her heart rate's down to 16,' and he said, 'That's not life, that's just reflex.'

"I held her for a bit," the father said, "and with my hand on

143

her head I could feel a little pulse through my fingers, and then the pulse stopped. The nurse listened for the heartbeat for a minute but didn't get any. But then the machine started showing bleeps again. She listened for another minute while the machine was bleeping. Incidentally," he said, in an aside, "it was sort of grotesque in a way. The way those machines work is that they take only two heartbeats and they project the time between them to a minute every time there's two heartbeats in a row. So she was jumping from a heartbeat of zero to a heartbeat of 120 a minute. The nurse was listening while these beeps were going on, and she couldn't hear anything. It was just the electronic noise in the machine causing these beeps.

"A nurse cannot pronounce somebody dead, so she called over a resident. He obviously—you could see from his face and body language that he didn't want to be the one to do this."

"The nurses were crying," said the mother, who could barely speak at this point.

"The nurses were crying," echoed her husband, "and a number of them had stayed past their shift to be with us and to say good-bye to our daughter."

The father remembers that when the resident walked over to pronounce death, "He was very stiff and he couldn't find his watch. And so I held out my hand with my watch on it for a minute. And it really caused my arm to ache. And he watched my watch and he officially said"—the father broke down, but then regained his composure—"in a forced even tone, 'I have listened for one minute, and I have not discerned any heartbeat.' Then he looked up at the clock and he said, '1:34,' and the nurse said, 'Yes.' Really it was about 1:40 at that time, and I had felt the last pulse at about 1:15."

For at least the next hour the couple stayed together in the nursery, with the mother sitting in one of the rocking chairs ubiquitous in NICUs, holding her dead first-born child. When staff members were finally able to take the baby's body from her mother, the body was cleaned up and then taken to the couple in the NICU's family room. "You know that little premie outfit I'd gotten as a gift? I finally got to dress her in it," the mother said.

What goes through a parent's mind at such a time? "Part of me couldn't believe it was happening. Part of me was just apologizing to her," the mother said, vainly attempting to choke back tears. "And I was feeling so bad for my husband, feeling so bad for my husband."

Said her husband: "I was feeling so badly for my wife that she had carried her, and she'd been so alive and kicking inside of her. And I was feeling so badly for our baby, that she never had a chance. I was also feeling at the same time that she was so beautiful."

"She was," said her mother. "She was beautiful."

"I guess I'd noticed just at the end," her father mumbled through tears, "I guess most of the time there'd been something on her feet or there'd been IVs on her feet and although sometimes I had touched her feet I hadn't noticed: I guess I noticed for the first time really that her little toe on her left foot was bent inward in exactly the same way that mine is. I don't know, that just touched me so much. I knew this was my little girl, but that cemented it beyond question that this was my little girl.

"I don't know," the father continued, sobbing, "I just felt this total sadness. I had so many plans for the things we were going to do together. There was so much I wanted to show her, just experience with her. And I was so much aware that she had only been alive a couple of weeks, and it had seemed so rotten, especially the last week with her on the Pavulon and being paralyzed and not being able to respond to things and not knowing whether she felt trapped. But a lot of the time I held her my mind was just blank. I had expected it to be racing. But in my grief things have just gone slowly."

CHAPTER 8

Hard Choices in the Nursery

The high-tech world of the intensive care nursery is initially as foreign as the surface of the moon to the families of most of the more than 230,000 infants who are born each year needing this care. Like most parents of premature or sick newborns, the couple whose baby died after living only twenty-three days knew almost nothing about neonatal intensive care before they found themselves in need of it for their baby girl. This ignorance is natural in a nation in which we take for granted normal childbirth and perfectly formed, healthy, term babies. No expectant parents, after all, think they will have a sick baby. While women worry during pregnancy about the things that might go wrong, such dark thoughts are usually saved for the middle of the night and don't intrude on the planning for labor, delivery and the decoration of the new nursery at home.

But the route from conception to an infant's arrival in a lovingly furnished nursery is not always smooth, and in recent years at least $2 billion has been spent annually in providing neonatal intensive care to about 230,000 babies in 600 intensive care nurseries in the United States. This money is spent without society asking whether it is buying $2 billion worth of benefit. There is no discussion about whether this care achieves acceptable outcomes. No congressman asks if this $2 billion could be better spent in some other area of health care. In what has traditionally been the American way of doing such things, physicians and hospital administrators simply act on the assumption that babies who can be saved should be saved. There is no public debate or discussion about how the bill will ultimately be paid.

In the past two decades it has become increasingly possible for neonatologists (pediatricians specializing in the care of newborns) to save smaller and smaller, and sicker and sicker infants. Perhaps nowhere in medicine have the improvements in survival been as dramatic as in the intensive care nursery (ICN), where care is provided for the 230,000 babies a year born weighing less than 2500 grams (5.5 pounds) as well as to those born with life-threatening birth defects and diseases. Two decades ago, nine out of ten babies born weighing less than 2.2 pounds died. Today, more than half survive. Indeed, in many of the 295 Level III ICNs, the most technologically and medically sophisticated of the intensive care nurseries, 75 percent of the babies weighing as little as one and a half pounds survive.

But keeping these babies alive is still no simple matter. It is the rare "premie" who does not suffer from one or more of the following problems: respiratory distress or failure, brain hemorrhages (which can cause retardation), pulmonary hemorrhages, inadequate sucking reflex, congestive heart failure, inadequate growth rate, fluid buildup around the heart, calcium deficiency and numerous infections. And not only is survival not a simple medical matter, it is not a cheap one either: Medical bills of upward of $150,000 are not uncommon for the tiniest of babies, those weighing less than 2.2 pounds, who may remain in ICNs for two, three, four or even nine months or more. While the low-income parents of many of these fetal infants are covered by Medicaid, the joint state-federal program of health insurance for the poor often pays as little as 27 cents on the dollar for neonatal care, forcing hospitals to raise their charges for other parents.

That means that the nation's insurers end up paying the bulk of the bills for this horrendously expensive care, which, in turn, means that all rate payers end up absorbing the costs as surely as they would if Medicaid paid and recovered the money through taxation.

Even when the available money is unlimited, it cannot always buy survival, or when it does, quality survival. Not many years ago, the intensive care nursery of a Washington, D.C., hospital cared for a pair of twins born prematurely at twenty-four weeks' gestation. One infant lived thirty-six hours. The other survived for three days. The cost of the fruitless effort to save them was $15,000. There are those who would argue that such efforts are an expensive waste. But who is to determine, at the moment of birth, that the effort should not be made to save two apparently perfect, albeit tiny, infants. Surely the parents of such infants would initially want everything done for them. And, when it looks like a normal outcome is at least possible, there aren't many neonatologists who are going to stand by and watch an infant die.

The question of "normal outcome" or, put another way, "quality survival," is highly charged, emotionally, ethically, legally and—with the advent of the "Baby Doe" cases in various hospitals around the country—politically. As we will discuss in greater detail in the next two chapters, probably at least once a day, in an ICN somewhere in the country, physicians and parents grapple with the question of whether the life of a sick newborn is worth saving. But even when the decision is made to go all out to save a sick premature newborn, caring physicians are still left wondering what kind of future they are saving such a child for. As Dr. William Silverman, former director of the nurseries at Babies Hospital in Manhattan, wrote in his book *Retrolental Fibroplasis: A Modern Parable:* "At Babies Hospital, I once reared a premature infant who weighted 800 grams [one pound, eight ounces] at birth. Three months and several tens of thousands of dollars after birth, the infant was sent home to a Harlem flat. Within a week, we heard that the infant died at night when a rat chewed off his nose."

And as parents struggle through the weeks and months of "roller coaster" existence, standing by as their baby struggles for life, they often ask themselves if they are doing the right thing. As twenty-two-year-old Lisa O'Riley put it, her voice choked by tears, "From where I am now, it would have been better if I miscarried. There's no way you can understand the kind of hell it's like living for three months not knowing if he's going to live, or if he's going to die, and if he does live, if he's ever going to know who you are."

Joey O'Riley was delivered at North Shore University Hospital in Manhasset, New York, weighing 910 grams, or about two pounds. About fourteen weeks premature, he was right on what might by today's standards be realistically called the border of viability. In fact, at the time of Joey's birth his mother was told he "had a ten- to twenty-percent chance of making it through the night"—and from there on it got worse. Specifically, it got worse because Joey O'Riley suffered a series of intraventricular hemorrhages (bleeding episodes in his brain) that caused severe brain damage. He developed hydrocephalus—a buildup of fluid in the brain—and eventually had to undergo six neurosurgical procedures. And, despite more than three months of hospitalization and bills in excess of $200,000, Lisa O'Riley ended up with a severely brain-damaged child who will never have anything approaching a normal life. But no one ever stopped and asked, "Should we be doing this? Is it right?" It was simply assumed that saving the life of a baby is the right thing to do. An ever-growing number of "premies" who are being treated are growing into young children who can only be called prisoners of technology, youngsters whose lungs were so damaged by disease and

149

the very machines used to save them that they cannot be removed from the machines. At Babies Hospital there was a two-year-old respirator-dependent child. Philadelphia Children's Hospital has a group of children it has discharged from the neonatal intensive care unit (NICU) to go home with respirators. North Shore University Hospital has had children in the nursery as long as a year, and infants who have finally been discharged only to go home depending upon machines for the very breaths keeping them alive.

In its final report, the now disbanded President's Commission for the Study of Ethical Problems in Medicine and Biomedical and Behavioral Research noted that: "Medicine's increased ability to forestall death in seriously ill newborns has magnified the already difficult task of physicians and parents who must attempt to assess which infants will benefit from various medical interventions, and which will not. Not only does this test the limits of medical certainty in diagnosis and prognosis, it also raises profound ethical issues."

What this comes down to is the fact that having the ability to save a grossly premature infant carries with it the responsibility to decide whether such a baby should be saved. Neonatologists are constantly forced to grapple with the question of when enough is enough. Improvements in neonatal survival in the past two decades have come about as a result of advances in technology and improvements in the understanding of fetal and neonatal physiology, improvements in the ability to provide nourishment to infants so premature they can legally be aborted as nonpersons.

Technological advances in neonatology usually occur piecemeal, with the improvement of a respirator here, a monitor there. Rarely do these advances appear on the scene in such a way that they have an immediate and profound impact on infant survival and the cost of that survival in the way that, say, CAT scanners have had on adult medicine. Now, however, such a new technology is being introduced into a still small but ever-increasing number of nurseries around the country. It is called extracorporeal membrane oxygenation, or ECMO, and its developers and supporters believe it can drastically improve neonatal survival and reduce long-term illness—at an added cost of from $1000 to $2000 a day for each day it is used. And that brings us to the stories of Erin Darlington and Shawn Myles.

Erin Darlington was delivered by cesarean section on June 9, 1983, sometime between the thirty-fourth and thirty-sixth week of her gestation. "There were no problems at the time of delivery," said Kathy Darlington, recalling her daughter's birth. "She had Apgar scores of eight and nine [which indicate excellent neurological and cardiovascular function] and she weighed five pounds and thirteen ounces. She was very healthy."

But by the end of her first hour of life, Erin was beginning to have difficulty breathing. She had developed idiopathic respiratory distress syndrome (IRDS), best known to the public as hyaline membrane disease, the most common killer of premature babies. The baby's condition worsened with each passing hour. "This was on a Thursday," her mother said, "and she proceeded to go downhill until Sunday."

At 5 A.M. on the Saturday after Erin Darlington's birth, Dr. Robert Bartlett entered Erin's mother's hospital room at the University of Michigan Hospital in Ann Arbor. "That entire night we couldn't sleep and had been up praying," Kathy Darlington recalled. "I was on pain medication and it was all a nightmare. There was no question when Dr. Bartlett presented the case what we should do. They'd tried everything. They'd been coming back and forth to see us. They'd say, 'We're going to try this now,' then they'd say, 'We're going to try that,' and of course we'd say yes. But they kept coming back and saying the procedures weren't working. It was emotionally draining, and I just wanted to hold my baby. I didn't think she was going to die,

B. D. COLEN

and when [my in-laws] started talking about what happens when
a baby dies, I didn't participate in the discussion."

What Bartlett told the Darlingtons was that he believed Erin
had only one chance at survival: that she be put on ECMO, the
experimental procedure that he has refined and applied to
humans. "Dr. Bartlett did point out some of the dangers," said
Erin's mother, "but at that point they were things that seemed
really small to us." So consent was given.

"She went through ECMO like a breeze," recalled Kathy
Darlington. "The first forty-five hours or so she didn't seem to
get better. But then she began to improve and they could turn
down the machine. . . . While she was on ECMO she woke up
and she appeared more healthy. She got pinker because her
blood was being oxygenated. You'd begin to think, 'Look at her.
She's fine.' And you'd forget the cannulas [tubes] coming out of
her neck and her groin. But you'd get to the point where you
wouldn't see them. I was there to let her know she had a mom,
and that these people sticking needles into her weren't her mom.
I did a lot of singing to her, and she still likes being sung to," said
Mrs. Darlington, who was with her daughter in the ICN at all
hours of the night and day. "I'd sing the second movement of
Beethoven's Pastoral and hymns. I remember singing 'Amazing
Grace' to her."

When Erin came off ECMO after sixty-five hours "it was a
victory. . . . Everyone was dancing around," Darlington recalled.
"They'd conquered death there. It was a true victory." Ten
months later, Erin Darlington is developing normally. "She's a
chubby little thing. She sits up, she says Dada—and she says that
to Dada," boasts her mother.

Would the Darlingtons be as happy with ECMO if they had
taken home a permanently damaged baby? "It would have de-
pended on the extent of how badly off she was," replied Erin's
mother. ". . . But I don't think that's a fair question." Maybe
not. But . . .

Shawn Myles's story began similarly. He was three weeks premature when he was delivered by cesarean section on July 12, 1982. He had an Apgar score of 8 at birth, but two minutes later he was experiencing respiratory distress and his score had dropped to 2. "I saw him when I came out of surgery," said Shawn's mother, Laura Myles. "They wheeled me into the intensive care nursery and he was on a respirator. He weighed seven pounds, ten ounces. He was the biggest baby in there. I was shocked, but I thought everything was going to be fine. At first they thought he had hyaline membrane disease, but they thought he'd be fine. They said, 'Just give him a couple of days.' "

But Shawn's condition, too, steadily deteriorated. Four days after his delivery, the physicians caring for him in Grand Rapids decided his only chance at life lay in a transfer to the neonatal intensive care unit at the University of Michigan Hospital in Ann Arbor. "From what they say now, he was very close to dying at that point," recalled Laura Myles. "But the way that some people talked, we were going to go down there and it was going to be a miracle." And indeed, it appeared to be so.

Shawn Myles was transferred to Ann Arbor specifically to be placed on ECMO. "But when we got to Ann Arbor there was already a baby on ECMO," said Laura Myles. "He was nine days old before they could get him on it. He had twelve chest tubes at one time or another, and his lungs were getting a lot worse. They were telling us that he wasn't a candidate for ECMO yet. I think they said that so we wouldn't feel bad. But as soon as they took the other baby off, Shawn was instantly put on it. They told us they would hook him up to it and there were no guarantees, but there was an eighty-percent survival rate, and if there was any bleeding in the brain they'd stop," the mother recalled. "At that point we felt it was the only thing that would save him." And, said Myles, she and her husband, Dan, also felt that turning off the machines and allowing Shawn to die would be the right thing to do if he suffered a serious hemorrhage in his brain.

Shawn was nine days old, "the oldest baby they'd put on ECMO," by the time the system was available to him. "He got off a lot faster than they thought he would," said his mother, "but he was still on [oxygen] afterwards. He was on oxygen until July [1983]. They said it looked like buckshot [holes] in his lungs," Laura Myles recalled, describing the lung damage apparently caused by the initial use of the respirator. Shawn spent two months in NICUs in Ann Arbor and Grand Rapids before finally being sent home. At first, his mother thought she had "a normal baby who would outgrow his lung problems." But by the following spring, she said, "I started questioning the doctor as to whether there was brain damage or not. . . . All he would say is, 'We won't know until he's older,' and 'he's got a lot of potential.' He still says that now."

As Shawn, whose care cost over $100,000, approached his second birthday, "he was at a seven- to thirteen-month level," his mother said. "He's a very alert little kid. He's very stubborn. He's just sitting up now. He's not eating real well. He drinks formula and we're just getting to where he'll eat baby food. He's real thin." And his medical problems were not yet over. "He was back in the hospital four times with pneumonia," his mother said. "He was in for a week this last month and that alone was six thousand dollars and that was only for six days." Between a good private insurance policy and the Michigan Crippled Children's program, Shawn's astronomical medical bills have been taken care of. But early on in his care, said his mother, "we had no idea what was going to be covered, and all we could think of was going bankrupt." In spite of her son's difficulties, Laura Myles said, "We feel that we would do it over again with the outcome we got." Even if it meant bankruptcy? "Yes," she replied, without hesitation.

When Erin Darlington and Shawn Myles were placed on ECMO it was classified as an investigational procedure, as it still was in the summer of 1985. Its use was and is not regulated by the federal or state governments but was and is limited to trials on a very small group of very sick newborns. "The babies this is done on have both feet in the grave," said Dr. Charles Stolar, a pediatric surgeon at Babies Hospital in New York City, which has an ECMO program. Indeed, at the majority of the more than dozen institutions setting up ECMO programs, the only babies being offered the new treatment are those who are believed to have less than a 20-percent chance of surviving with conventional treatment. At both Children's Hospital National Medical Center in Washington, D.C., and North Shore University Hospital on Long Island, the first babies to go on ECMO were those with less than a 10-percent chance of survival without it.

Despite its fancy acronym, this theoretically life-saving procedure involves little more than the ever-so-carefully monitored use of a form of heart-lung machine. It is really a quite simple device, consisting of some plastic tubing, a pump and a gas-permeable membrane. The tubing is surgically inserted into a vein and an artery in the infant's body, and the oxygen-depleted blood is pumped out of the body, through the membrane, where it is oxygenated, and back into the body. The rationale for the procedure is that it will give the infant's overworked heart and damaged or underdeveloped lungs a chance to rest and repair themselves while the ECMO system does its work, just as a bypass pump carries a patient through open-heart surgery. And even to an educated layperson, the rationale sounds reasonable.

At this point, the procedure's use is generally limited to three groups of full-term infants: those with diaphragmatic hernias, a condition in which intestine has collected in the chest cavity and prevented full lung development; those with persistent fetal circulation, in whom blood is shunted from one side of the heart to the other—as it should be in the fetus—without passing through the lungs for oxygenation; and those with severe meconium aspiration, a condition in which fetal feces have accumulated in the lungs. What so excites neonatologists about ECMO is that initial statistics from Robert Bartlett's group at Michigan suggest that infants with less than a 20-percent chance of surviving with current treatment have a 90-percent chance of surviving with ECMO. Asked if it wasn't a difficult decision to place a sick newborn on ECMO, Dr. Rita Harper, chief of neonatology at North Shore and an associate professor of perinatal medicine at Cornell University Medical College, replied: "That's not a hard choice: The kid's going to die if you don't do it."

But as Dr. Billie Short, the neonatologist running the ECMO program at Children's Hospital National Medical Center, points out, "the reality of ECMO is there will be some babies surviving because of ECMO that may have severe brain damage." This damage, caused by the baby's underlying disease, is often undetectable before the baby goes on ECMO. These babies, she notes, are not surviving now despite an "all stops out [effort] . . . using every drug we have."

Were the use of ECMO limited to the saving of a few categories of babies in a handful of highly sophisticated institutions, its use might never represent a hard choice. But there are already indications that the use of ECMO will spread, and spread quickly—before there are any properly controlled clinical trials to test its medical usefulness, and before any cost-benefit analysis is done to see if the use of ECMO can reduce hospital stays and costs. And at least one pioneer in the care of newborns sees in the very introduction of ECMO the potential for a disaster of enormous proportions.

Following the introduction into the newborn nursery of high concentrations of life-saving oxygen, thousands of babies were blinded by a condition called retrolental fibroplasia (RLF), which

156

is believed to be caused by the action of oxygen upon the blood vessels of the newborn's eyes. Between 1941, when the first case was noted, and 1954, some 10,000 cases of blindness were attributed to RLF and all of those, says Dr. William Silverman, who lived through the RLF debacle as chief of the nurseries at Babies Hospital, were avoidable. Known as the "father" of modern neonatology, Silverman retired from active practice because of what he saw as a lack of good science in perinatal medicine. Too many treatments, he believed, were being introduced without properly controlled trials. ECMO, he says, "is history repeating itself. Once you say you're introducing a new treatment and you're just getting a pilot experience and later on you'll test it in a controlled fashion," there's no turning back. The initial "successful" experience will be used, he believes, as a rationale for never doing proper trials. Patients should have a chance to either be given or be protected from the new treatment. "When there are those who are eligible and meet your criteria, then do it in an organized fashion. Also," he warned, "this is oxygenating a newborn infant and we do not know the role of oxygen in causing retrolental fibroplasia. . . . History would show you that when you're oxygenating a newborn you should do so cautiously. I'm quite convinced this is a very interesting approach, just on theoretical terms," he continued. "But the next step is to test it in a responsible fashion, and responsible means it has been subjected to rigorously controlled trials. Good science means you protect people's rights. You don't say, 'Oops, sorry.' You do things in such a way as to minimize risks."

But what of the apparently excellent first results being achieved with ECMO? "Nothing works so well as a treatment without concurrent controls," Silverman replied, suggesting that the only way to know if ECMO really saves lives is to alternately give it to and withhold it from a set number of babies who qualify for it.

Questions of controls aside, ECMO is a highly labor-intensive technology, requiring the involvement of surgeons, neonatologists, nurses and technicians. Any institution establishing an ECMO program should have an animal research laboratory to enable it to run trials on newborn sheep before using the system on humans. And the hospital needs enough neonatal admissions to make the establishment of a program cost-efficient. While Dr. Dietrich Roloff, chief of neonatology at Michigan and a man directly involved in the ECMO work there, says he sees the possible need for an ECMO "network on the order of magnitude of one per state," there are already several ECMO programs in California, there is one on Long Island and one in Manhattan forty minutes away, there is one at Children's in Washington, and Georgetown University Medical Center in the same city is planning a program—all before the word is in on the ultimate value of the technology. Told of Roloff's statement that ECMO should be limited to a handful of institutions, Dr. John Scanlon, chief of neonatology at Columbia Hospital for Women in Washington, laughed. "Sure," he said, "just like CAT scans patients, but you can bet your bottom dollar that if private industry puts a lot of dollars in this it's not going to end up as an 'orphan drug' [a life-saving remedy that can benefit too few patients to be economically practicable]." Not only is it unlikely that ECMO will be abandoned once its use spreads, it is also unlikely that its use will continue to be limited to a small number of patients.

If ECMO was used only for term babies for whom there is no other treatment, and if it proves as useful as Bartlett's initial results suggest it may be, it would probably slip into general use with few questions asked. After all, while ECMO may raise the cost of neonatal intensive care to over $3000 a day, it is expected babies will be on the machine for fewer than ten days, and in some cases as few as two. And while $30,000 isn't cheap, without ECMO those same babies might be in an ICN for three or more months, at a cost of well over $100,000, and they might then go home with permanent lung damage, brain damage and other serious problems. What worries some neonatologists, however, is that once hospitals have ECMO, they will begin using it on smaller and smaller premature infants, eventually using it to try to save the babies weighing as little as one pound. While it is not yet technically possible to save such a tiny "premie" with ECMO, Short at Children's Hospital thinks "there are all kinds of ethical decisions that have to be made. The 1000- or 800- grammer at this stage is already in our nurseries a long time," Short said. "It would have to be shown effective before it should be allowed to be used on these babies. There would have to be a very defined research protocol to be able to say we are in effect decreasing the hospital stay for these babies."

Michigan's Robert Bartlett does not advocate rushing into the generalized use of ECMO. "There are several things that lead us to not pursuing this as yet in the infant, say, between 500 and 1000 grams, but they're not technical—it could be done— they're primarily ethical and allocation-of-resources issues," said the professor of surgery. "This is a new technique that's under study, and we think we should learn all about it and find out if it's useful in the full-term baby first, and if it's useful in that group, then it's worth expending the dollars and effort to evaluate it in the smaller infant. If it isn't going to work in big babies it sure isn't going to work in small babies."

But when ECMO was first conceived of a decade ago, it was part of a scheme to produce an artificial placenta, allowing fetal development to take place outside the womb for women who could not carry a baby to term. And, said Bartlett, "it's not too far a jump to think about test-tube conception and growing the entire fetus in an in vitro system. I'm not suggesting doing that, but we're obviously doing test-tube conceptions many places in the country and putting the embryo back in the uterus and letting it grow. Somewhere there's a jump between that and attaching it to the blood supply, but beginning with a full-term baby and working backwards you could get to the point of taking a very premature fetus and supporting it in an extracorporeal environment," in which the fetus would float in warm liquid, with machines providing its blood oxygenation and dialyzing its kidneys.

In 1983 the *New England Journal of Medicine* published a study by a group of researchers on the business and medical faculties at McMaster University in Hamilton, Ontario, entitled "Economic Evaluation of Neonatal Intensive Care of Very-Low-Birth-Weight Infants." The researchers at McMaster were analyzing—in a cold-blooded way—the economic impact of the institution of a system of regionalized neonatal care in Ontario, but their findings can be generalized to the American setting. In terms of the cost of years of life gained by providing neonatal care—taking into account long-term health care costs and potential future earnings of the infants—caring for babies in the 1500- to 1000-gram category was cost-effective. But when the high-tech, personnel-intensive care was given to infants weighing less than 1000 grams, the result was a net economic loss.

As John Scanlon points out, "society has always been willing to pay for loss leaders," either out of humanitarian interest or because there is a promise of future benefits, like an investment, and that's exactly what neonatal intensive care is. "We're now taking kids of 1500 grams for granted [in that they do so well] and there's a ripple effect." Scanlon and many other physicians who have thought about these kinds of issues insist that it's not up to physicians like themselves to decide whether programs like ECMO are too expensive. "It's society's problem, but society's been unwilling to deal with it," he said. Society, not physicians at the bedside, must choose where it wants its health dollars spent. While we cannot go on spending apparently limitless amounts of money in every area of medical endeavor, says Scanlon, society, not physicians, must decide where to apply the brakes. "There's a finite number of dollars," he continued. "But society hasn't been willing to deal with this in adult medicine because everybody says, 'Hell, it may be me that keels over with all my coronaries gone.' It's easy to make these decisions in the newborn: 'It's okay, dear, you can always have another baby.' 'Well, he would have been brain-damaged anyway.' 'They're dumb and they're poor, and what the hell, they'll go out and spawn again anyway.' Look, that's where these things are tested anyway," he said, referring to new technologies and treatment methods. "They're not being tested in white middle-class America, they're tested in teaching hospitals, and who goes to the teaching hospitals? So we test things there and then the question is, do they get exported to the suburbs, and if so to whom, and who's going to bear the cost for it? And those aren't medical issues. It's unfair to expect medicine to shoulder the responsibility for that.

"The problem," Scanlon said, "is that in this society we regulate our health care costs on the basis of population statistics, but we make our decisions on an individual basis. . . . This society, like a lot of ethicists, is wonderful at analysis not only after the horse has been stolen, but after the barn's been burned. Getting the answer is easy, it's the application of the answers that's difficult."

V.
THE BABIES DOE

CHAPTER 9
Nobody Looks at Cara Lynn

When Bob and Marty Bailey go for a walk, strangers often approach to take a peek at what's inside the Perego twin stroller that Marty pushes along in front of her. "They always come up and say, 'Oh, let me see the ba—' and they blanch and turn away," Bob said.

Nearly everyone does blanch at the first sight of Bob and Marty's daughter, Cara Lynn. Bob himself just "stood there and cried" the first time he saw Cara. But then, what parent, or what person for that matter, is prepared for the first view of what the dictionary describes as an "anencephalic monster," an infant born with no cerebral cortex and, in Cara's case, a skull that looks as though it has been sawed off about two inches above eyelids that are fused shut?

When Bob and Marty saw their child the first time after her birth, they didn't even notice many of Cara's other deformities.

They noticed the cleft lip, which opens all the way into her right nostril. They could see the hollow eye sockets, covered with the fused lids and extraordinarily lush lashes. They could see that her ears didn't match and were set too low on her head.

But she was wearing a hospital cap, so they couldn't see the fluid-filled, bluish and mottled pink membrane covering the top of her head. And she was wrapped in a blanket, so they couldn't see that some of her fingers were fused together and some were missing. They couldn't tell that one arm was functionally no more than a flipper. They were unaware that she had a mal-formed clavicle and a deformed hip. They wouldn't see the de-formed toes and club foot until they later unwrapped the blanket. They had no way of knowing that, in fact, the only symmetrical parts of her body were her two perfectly formed thumbs.

And they didn't know then that she was alive only in the most rudimentary sense, unable ever to function on more than a re-flexive, primitive, nonsentient level.

Marty Bailey says she knew early in her pregnancy that some-thing was wrong with the fetus she was carrying, but she couldn't convince her obstetrician. "I asked the doctor for a son-ogram," she said, sitting on the couch in the living room of her suburban home. "But he said no, it wasn't his standard practice. All my friends had pictures of their babies in utero. I was sure I was carrying her too low. All my friends carried their babies high, they all had trouble breathing. And one arm felt like a flip-per, not an arm, when it moved."

But Marty's doctor told her it wasn't standard practice in his office to provide ultrasound imaging for women her age—she was twenty-seven at the time—without a specific indication, and a mother's "feeling" was not a good enough indication. "I really did feel like I was carrying low," Marty said, "but when he said it was within the range of normal, I thought that he knew better."

Except for little "telltale signs" that Marty couldn't quite ar-ticulate, the pregnancy went along normally, she said, "until one week into the eighth month when I hemorrhaged."

"I was getting ready to go to work in the morning," she said. "I was getting dressed and all of a sudden I had a gush of blood." Bob was already at his job in the catering department of an airline when Marty called, telling him she was going to the hospital. A neighbor drove Marty to the hospital and the obstetrician met her there.

"They prepped me for delivery," she recalled. "They sent me down for a sonogram and they took a long time with the sonogram and then they put me back in the room." After the sonogram the doctor met with Bob, who had arrived at the hospital. "He said if he was going to send somebody for an ultrasound he wouldn't send them there, but keeping that in mind, he said that there could be one of two things: The baby could have a cyst or it could have hydrocephalus."

The physician said he wanted clarification and confirmation of the finding, and so the next morning he sent Marty to an ultrasonographer outside the hospital. The ultrasonographer had no sooner completed the exam than he told the couple to return immediately to their obstetrician. "He told us things did not look good," Marty said. "He told us that the baby had severe hydrocephalus and they didn't think she'd live."

"His phrase," said Bob, who will always remember the exact words, "was 'incompatible with life.'"

"He put me on bed rest and tranquilizers," Marty said. "Everybody asked me why he wasn't inducing labor, they asked why I had to go through those three weeks knowing what was coming at the end." The couple did "a lot of crying, a lot of crying in those days," Marty said.

"I just sat at home," she said. "I hemorrhaged more than once. I just sat and did jigsaw puzzles. I did two of them. We'd sit down at the end of a day and start talking and we'd end up crying. It felt like forever waiting."

There was an inordinate amount of waiting, for Marty went ten days past her due date, expecting to deliver a dead or dying baby, before she finally went into labor. And when she went to the hospital that April morning, all she could think of was that "we were going to have a baby and the baby was going to die."

"But we knew we were going to go through something that a lot of other people had gone through, and we knew we'd make it," Bob added.

Marty had arrived at the hospital at 10:30 in the morning, and by mid-afternoon her contractions were still mild and far apart. At that point the obstetrician did his first internal exam. "I heard a 'hmmmmmmmm,'" Bob recalled. "I said, 'Hmmmmmmmm what?' He said, 'I think we've got a problem.' I said, 'What problem?' and he said, 'I don't know what I'm feeling.'" Even after having an X-ray taken, the physician was still unsure what he was seeing. He even told Bob that he thought the X-ray had been taken wrong because, Bob recalled being told, "'the top of the baby's head is missing.'" But when the obstetrician called in a radiologist for a second opinion on the X-ray, he and Bob and Marty learned that there was nothing wrong with the X-ray: The baby Marty was carrying was indeed missing the top of its head. It was anencephalic, not hydrocephalic. "These terms didn't mean anything to us at the time," Bob said. "The death part did, but nothing else."

Marty was given drugs to hasten delivery and quickly lost control of her contractions. She was then given general anesthesia, and the obstetrician told Bob to go home—the couple only lived about eight minutes from the hospital—promising to call as soon as anything happened. And about 8:30 P.M., only forty-five minutes after Bob had gotten home, "the phone rang and I picked it up and it was a doctor on the line and he said, 'I'm just calling you to tell you, first of all, that Marty's okay. You've had a baby girl and she's severely affected.' So he said, 'Come on up. We're getting your wife all cleaned up and I'll meet you in the delivery room.' He met me at the door and he said they're cleaning Marty up, but would you like to see the baby?" Bob remembered saying he would and then the doctor walking him down to the nursery area.

"One section was the nursery where they display all the kids and the other was the intensive care nursery," he said. "We didn't go in, but he walked up to me and put his arm around my shoulder and motioned for the nurse to bring the bassinet forward, because she was sort of stuck in the back of the room by herself. And that's when I saw her for the first time, and she was definitely a fearful, disturbing little thing to behold. Not to mention different than anything I'd ever seen. I'd seen kids with cleft lips before, but naturally never my own. He was very supportive and quite strong for me. And I stood there and cried and really felt really bad for her.

"But at the same time I wasn't emotionally involved with her other than to know that she was mine. There was a kind of detachment there because I couldn't see getting to know her to have her taken away from me. The next thing I said was, 'Now I'd like to see my wife.' "

Bob said he didn't pause to take stock of Cara's various deformities because he knew he was going to see her again when Marty came down for the first time and, more important, he did not want to become attached to a baby whom he had been told was going to die.

Bob's belief that Cara would die shortly was based on what he and Marty had been told about her having hydrocephalus making her incompatible with life. He didn't know at the time that children with hydrocephalus can live for years, if not decades. Nor did he know that anencephalics rarely leave the hospital alive, with most dying of infection within days of birth.

Marty recalled that when she came to after the delivery she "wasn't really told anything."

"I don't remember what I was told about what her condition was," the mother said, "just that she wasn't going to live for more than a day or two. I didn't really know what her problems were until I went down myself the next day. The doctor was there and he put his arm around me as well, he was very supportive, very kind through the whole thing, and they had her in a little isolette when I saw her, all the way back in the intensive care nursery. She was all covered up, I couldn't see her arms or legs or anything. She had the cap on. So I could barely see her. I kept telling them, 'Bring her closer, I can't see her.' They'd bring her a couple of inches, and I'd say, 'Closer.' They brought her up to the front and I started to cry, but I still couldn't really see her. I didn't really notice what was wrong with her at that time, until we got to see her more."

Marty was discharged from the hospital within twenty-four hours of the delivery, and she and Bob went home to be together. Bob had been told to make funeral arrangements for Cara, whose name had been picked out long before her delivery. The couple had told the physicians at the Catholic hospital that they didn't want any extraordinary means or any technology used to extend Cara's life. "I had the impression that my wife was the living one and Cara was going to be the dying one," Bob said, explaining that he somehow had been led to believe that Cara's death was assured, "but I don't know where I got that impression." But for two days the couple was told not to visit their daughter, not to get attached. They'd call to check on her condition and be told there was no change.

Finally, they could stand it no longer, said Bob, and they went to visit her for the first time. Then, as the days became weeks, the couple at first began visiting every two days, and then every day. They were becoming attached in spite of themselves. They'd read Cara's chart when they went in and would note that on some shifts she didn't seem to be getting her regular feedings, feedings that often took more than two hours because her cleft lip made it impossible for her to suck properly. "We'd ask them, 'Does this mean that you didn't feed her, or you just didn't put it down?' 'Oh, we just didn't put it down,'" Marty recalled being told.

"It never really became evident that she would make it," Marty said. After all, there was no record of an anencephalic ever living to six months. But as time passed the couple began to think about bringing their daughter home. "What got us to think about bringing her home was not that she was going to make it but because of the way that she was treated in the hospital," Marty said.

"We were starting to come away from the hospital and have discussions about what condition we'd find her in," Bob said, "meaning that she was neglected, or the way she was dressed; we'd find her naked, we'd find her propped in the bassinet only she'd slipped all the way to the bottom. We'd go in there and hear a little grunt under the blanket and she was in there." There were certainly signs that the infant was not receiving optimum care. She would be left in a room by herself, unchecked, for at least an hour at a time. She was moved from room to room on almost a daily basis in the pediatrics unit. When she got a staph infection she was quarantined—in a room with an open window. "We were coming home from the hospital and instead of feeling good that we'd just seen her, we'd be aggravated about the care. We were starting to get ticked off," said Bob, who was the first to suggest that it might be time to consider taking Cara home.

During one hospital visit, when the couple was alone with Cara, she began to cry. Marty had held her before, but had never picked her up. "Up until that time we'd always been handed her, but a doctor or a nurse would pick her up and put her in our arms," Bob said. "Marty said, 'I don't know what to do, I don't want to get a nurse in here just 'cause she's crying, I feel like I should be holding her.' So I said, 'Okay, hold her,' and I picked her up and put her in her arms. I couldn't damage her anymore than she was damaged already. I wasn't going to drop her, I felt pretty secure in that. So 'Here's your daughter, take her.' I wasn't scared about it, I felt like she's mine, and that, I think,

171

was the turning point. I said if there's no apparent change in six weeks, let's take her home."

"I was more tired out going back and forth to the hospital than I would be if she was here," Marty said.

The end of the hospital stay finally came when Bob and Marty arrived one day to visit Cara and found her lying in a bassinet, a bottle propped in her mouth, choking on formula that was spilling down her face. The next day the couple took their daughter home. "We decided that if she was going to live eight weeks, twelve weeks, whatever extraordinary time, she deserved a life of love with her parents, not in the hands of detached professionals. We decided to have a baby and we had a baby," Bob said.

While bringing Cara home may have been "best" for Cara, assuming that she could benefit from more loving care—and that is a big assumption—it condemned Marty to what she could only describe a year and a half later as a life of "shift work." Marty had decided to speak with me then because she was so outraged by the much publicized Baby Doe case on Long Island, a case in which the Reagan administration, spurred on by so-called right-to-life organizations, was fighting to obtain the medical records of a deformed infant at a local hospital. "There's nobody to help me," she said then. "Where are they?" she asked of the people who would force parents and physicians to save every infant, no matter how damaged. "They step into a life, do their thing and good-bye. . . . These people save a life, clap their hands after it's done and then they turn away."

Ironically, at the same time the administration was fighting unsuccessfully to force surgery for one defective infant, the Baileys were fighting to convince Medicaid that they deserved help for Cara. On his $40,000 annual income—including overtime—there was no way Bob could hire nursing care for the baby. And without nurses, Marty couldn't go back to work. In fact, without nurses, Marty couldn't do anything but care for Cara twenty-four hours a day. The infant's head dressings, which cost more than $600 a month, had to be changed every two hours. She had to be spoon-fed every three hours. Her diapers had to be changed constantly, as they would for the rest of her life. Marty couldn't find baby-sitters who were either willing or capable of caring for the infant. On the few occasions when the parents tried to hire a licensed practical nurse to care for Cara, the woman would generally leave after one shift and never return. Bob Bailey said that in his frustration he wrote to the White House and "invited Ronnie Reagan into our house.

"We said, 'Come on down, step right up, take a look at reality. If you can care for her, then you can tell me what to do.' We even sent pictures of her," Bob said. "He never even acknowledged it. That son of a bitch never even sent us an autographed picture thanking us for the support we never gave him.

"What he was doing to the Does he did to us," said Bob, who then laughed and added, "We were offering them the chance of a lifetime! How many people get a chance to meet somebody like her?" He gestured toward the middle of the living room, where his by then four-and-a-half-year-old daughter lay on her back on a wheelchair. She was doing what she always did, and would do as long as she lived. Her arms were in slow motion, her fused fingers now brushing over her size 4-T flowered sundress, now probing her gaping hole of a mouth, now rubbing, rubbing at her forehead, as if to push away pain. Marty rose from the couch and picked Cara up, and then sat back down, with Cara's head on her arm and the rest of her three-foot-long body draped across Marty's lap in a Pietà-like position.

Medicaid did finally agree to help the Baileys, but only after they threatened to institutionalize Cara, which the government would have had to pay for and which would be far more expensive than home care. But under a ruling known as the Katie Beckett exception, the program will pay for home care in cases where the parents aren't poor enough to normally qualify for Medicaid if the alternative is for the child to be made a ward of the state and be institutionalized. Of course, during the eighteen months Medicaid was denying Bob and Marty help, no one ever mentioned the Katie Beckett exception. It wasn't until Marty talked to the right person at the right self-help group that she learned about it. And so Marty's nightmare life of captivity ended after about nineteen months. At that point Medicaid agreed the couple was entitled to eight hours of RN care for Cara each day, at $120 a shift. The couple elected to have nurses come in only five days a week, to preserve some sense of privacy in their home, but even at that, Cara's nursing bills alone come to $31,200 a year, more than Bob's base gross salary. And with the special gauze for her head, at $400 a case, plus underpads, other dressings and diapers, her supplies come to well over $1000 a month. So federal and state taxpayers are paying well over $43,-000 a year to maintain the life of a child who has no self-awareness, let alone an ability to receive and return love.

Despite all this, Bob and Marty Bailey love their daughter, and this creates enormous dilemmas for them. On the one hand, they say she and they will be far better off when she dies. On the other, the one time she had serious respiratory difficulties at home, they immediately called the pediatrician for medication. But on the single occasion when fluid began to leak through the inflated membrane covering her brain, the couple said they just "sat here and we watched as her head collapsed, totally collapsed," in Bob's words.

"We didn't call the doctor or anything," he said. "We didn't do anything other than make ourselves a drink and watch it deflate, and it literally deflated. It looked like a cup that the contents spilled out of. The outer membrane of her head just flattened as flat as a puddle of liquid. And her head actually looked like a vessel that had emptied its contents. We stood and waited for the end. But it didn't come. She got happier and happier. We put her to bed that night and said, 'Well, if we wake up and she's dead, that's it.' But we didn't call the doctor. We didn't try to take a Band-Aid and plug the leak or anything. We had been told that when that happened to her, that would be the end for her: cerebral fluid, puddle, bingo! Death. End of story." But it wasn't the end of the story. For the leaking fluid simply relieved pressure building up in Cara's skull, and rather than become infected and die, she apparently became more comfortable.

How can the parents rationalize calling the pediatrician if their child has difficulty breathing, but not helping her if her head springs a leak? They simply say that they will treat normally those conditions any child would normally get. If Cara has difficulty breathing, a problem that is not related to her deformities, they will treat her just as they would treat their normal child. But if her life is threatened by a problem related to her condition, they will not treat it. They said they would not, for instance, ever start tube-feeding for her should it become "necessary" at some point in the future.

But when Marty was asked if infants like Cara should be starved at birth, she replied, "I certainly don't think all the time she's spent has been the best, but I can't say myself that I could not give her food because obviously I did when I brought her home. I took care of her because she's my daughter. I couldn't see her starve to death, I couldn't see her in that kind of pain, and I've heard that that's painful, so I couldn't say that the hospital staff should do that either, because they're human beings who would only have to watch her die the same way. So I can't say that she shouldn't have been fed, but maybe if she had just not eaten on her own, it would have been because she had the cleft lip, and she couldn't have eaten as much and then she wouldn't have gained weight and she would have died a lot earlier. That might have been kinder than to see her come this far."

175

"But we've often talked about the fact we couldn't make that decision to end her life, that's not my decision to make," Bob said. "She's lived this far because she's lived this far, not because we've sustained her. And that's not a religious view, we're not religious people in any formal way. But at the same time, I couldn't withhold something from her. It would have been kinder if she had died. She hasn't lived a life, she's had an existence, one filled with pain, a lot of suffering and, yeah, I'd much rather not have gone through this whole thing. Had we known in enough time and been given the choice, I think we would have aborted her. . . ."

"That would have been the optimum," Marty interrupted, "because then nobody would have suffered. But since she was born, to take food away from her"—she shook her head. "She's lived on her own. If the whole thing could have been avoided, that would have been better. . . ." But then she thought for a minute again about the question of starving such newborns, and began, "I feel like, looking back, if she could have been made comfortable—"

Bob interrupted, somewhat incredulous, "You could say that, Marty? That you could withhold nourishment? You could say that?"

"Yes," said Marty, who had been up with Cara every three hours, every night, for the past four and a half years. "Yes," said Marty, who, after delivering a second, normal baby, had to care for both Cara and her new son around the clock without help. "Yes," said Marty, who spends at least ten hours a day with Cara, trying to care for a normal child as well, while Bob is at work. "Yes, I don't believe in making that kind of decision, but in a case like hers, it's not just a quality-of-life issue with me, it's not just that she's just lying there. But she's gone through a lot. She's in pain. I don't want to think about taking her life away because that is a big thing, but yet, she wouldn't have suffered all that time either, and I've seen that for four and a half years."

Should society be paying to sustain lives like Cara's? the couple was asked.

"Given the option she wouldn't be here," Bob said. "So obviously we feel. . . . Even in spite of having her, if she were to die tonight, it would be a very, very big loss, because we're attached to her, but at the same time it would be the best possible thing for everybody, including her, and us. I couldn't put a dollar-and-cents value on it. Obviously she's cost a lot of people a lot of money, including us, and a lot of sweat, and all that, but financially I couldn't use that as a reason, but there's no doubt about the fact that she shouldn't be here. Whether it cost somebody one dollar or fifty cents or a million dollars, nobody should have to pay the burden of a baby like her because she shouldn't be here, and again, if we were given our choice, she wouldn't be here. . . ."

"But you can't put into words, or legislation, what should be done," Marty said.

"We love her enough to let her go," Bob said, "which to me is the supreme kind of love. We're not to the point of loving her so much that we want her to live a life that I can't really consider a life. She's living an existence. She had nothing to see. She has no idea who her parents are. She just knows us by touch, and that's just assumption on our part."

They think about how they will react when she dies.

"It will be very sad," Marty concluded, "and it will be a great relief."

CHAPTER 10

Premies and Politics

From the moment of her birth, Cara Lynn Bailey was a candidate for infanticide. In fact, it is not an exaggeration to say that what is surprising is not that she might have been killed but that she was not. "Somebody didn't do his job," a noted neonatologist said angrily when told about Cara. "She should never have left the delivery room." Indeed, it is not at all uncommon when a baby like Cara is born for the physician to place the infant in a tray in a corner of the delivery room and simply cover the tray with a towel and walk away. In a short time the infant is dead and the parents are told that the mother delivered a stillborn, badly malformed infant.

Dr. Julius Korein, professor of neurology at New York University and chief of the EEG labs at New York University–Bellevue Hospital, has often told the story of delivering a "monster" during his residency. "The woman gave birth to twins," Korein recalled. "One was normal and one was a monster. It looked like a bird: it had claws for hands and it had a beak. I didn't suction it, and I placed it in a pan and covered it. One of the nurses started to go over to it and I said, 'Don't touch it. I'll take care of it.' A few hours later I went back and it was dead. I told the parents that there had been twins but one had been born dead."

Throughout recorded history, and undoubtedly earlier, babies with birth defects have been killed or left to die. While we can all probably recall an elementary school teacher telling us in sonorous tones that the Spartans left deformed infants on mountainsides, we were less likely to be told, or to remember from our reading, that Plato's *Republic,* one of the philosophical blueprints of Western civilization, advocates killing defective newborns.

Definitions of "defective" have varied widely from period to period, civilization to civilization, even from parent to parent. To the ancient Greeks, any infant with a debilitating birth defect of any sort was a candidate for infanticide. In Germany of 1940 a baby with a Jewish mother was termed "defective," as was any infant or adult who was crippled or retarded, for that matter. In almost all civilizations during hard times, excess infants, who create a strain on limited resources, are treated as disposable defectives. Until very recently, certain peoples, including the Chinese, killed female babies at will.

It is only a combination of economic security and modern medical technology that has given today's "civilized" societies the luxury of vigorously seeking to protect the severely deformed from what is actually part of the process of natural selection. But as medical skill and technology have developed to the point where infants with major birth defects can be saved, parents and physicians have been forced for the first time to confront the difficult choice of whether or not to save severely deformed newborns. After all, it was not necessary to debate the morality of denying life-sustaining or life-prolonging surgery to infants with Down's syndrome when such surgery was unlikely to succeed. But with the refinement of pediatric surgical techniques, particularly in the area of cardiac surgery, it has become possible to save infants who could never before have been saved.

Thus, we are now confronted with the question of whether the infant with Down's syndrome should be treated any differently from the normal infant. Should information about the infant's potential IQ and quality of life play a part in the decision-making process when life itself is at stake? Should parents, who will have to raise and care for the defective child, be the ones who ultimately decide if the child should live or die?

Such decision making has become a given in the practice of neonatology, the care of sick and premature newborns. It is such a given that, in the fall of 1983, at the height of the Baby Doe controversy, Milwaukee neonatologist Stephen C. Ragatz was willing to be quoted as saying, "I've been in practice now for seventeen months and I have personally disconnected the respirator on youngsters three times." It has been estimated, in fact, that at least once a day, in one of the nation's more than 500 intensive care nurseries, life-prolonging care is withheld or withdrawn from an infant whose parents and physician have reluctantly decided that such care would not ultimately benefit the baby.

Traditionally, such decision making has been the province of parents and physicians acting, privately and in concert, in what they presume to be the best interests of the child. Errors in judgment do occur, and while such errors can lead to the death of a baby, those who err usually do so on the side of caution. In the first place, most parents want their baby to live, no matter how badly damaged or deformed. And it has been and continues to be extremely unusual for a physician to refuse to care for a damaged newborn whom a parent wants saved. Additionally, while neonatologists tend to be risk takers, they tend to take their risks in favor of life, always believing there is "just one more thing" that can be done, one more intervention that may turn the trick. One only need skim Robert and Peggy Stimson's harrowing book, *The Long Dying of Baby Andrew*, to quickly conclude that far more infants probably suffer needlessly in the name of vitalism than die of neglect as a result of parental selfishness or fear.

As business has traditionally been conducted in the nation's delivery rooms and intensive care nurseries, both parents and physicians have always had the option of turning to the legal system if they were unable to resolve disagreements over the appropriateness of treatment or nontreatment. While parents rarely, if ever, took doctors to court to get them to halt treatment or to force them to continue it, physicians were very much aware of the possibility that parents might later bring malpractice charges in civil court, certainly a check on physician authoritarianism. And physicians have long had and exercised the option of seeking a court order to compel treatment in cases where they disagreed with a parent's refusal to allow it.

There were three events in the early 1970s that began a decade of discussion and debate about the withholding of care from dying or badly deformed or retarded newborns.

One of these was the production of a film about a 1971 case in which a Down's syndrome infant at Johns Hopkins Hospital was allowed to starve to death rather than undergo relatively routine surgery to correct a duodenal atresia—a congenital lack of connection between stomach and intestine—a not uncommon complication of Down's syndrome. The film, a dramatization of the case and discussion of the issues involved, was and continues to be shown to audiences of professionals and laypersons interested in ethical issues and the care of newborns. Interestingly, while a decade ago there were a number of ethicists and neonatologists who were willing to publicly defend the position taken in the "Hopkins case," that is, the parents' decision to allow the infant to starve simply because it had Down's syndrome, when the same film was shown a decade later to a room full of neonatologists and nurses specializing in neonatal care, there was only one person in the room, a neonatologist, who raised his hand when asked if anyone agreed that the parents even had the right to make the decision they did. Certainly public airing of these issues over the course of a decade has resulted in a heightened awareness of the need to protect those who are simply mentally or physically handicapped, as opposed to infants who are doomed to meaningless lives of pain and nonawareness.

The second event that brought ethical issues of newborn care into the public arena was the publication in 1973 in the *New England Journal of Medicine* of the now famous Duff-Campbell article. Entitled "Moral and Ethical Dilemmas in the Special-Care Nursery," the article was a report on 299 consecutive deaths in the intensive care nursery of Yale–New Haven Hospital between 1970 and 1972, forty-three of which were the immediate result of a joint parent-physician decision to withdraw or withhold treatment. The authors of that study, Dr. Raymond S. Duff of Yale and Scottish physician Alexander G. M. Campbell, argued eloquently that there are times it is as wrong to attempt to prolong the life of a seriously deformed, or dying, newborn as it is to fail to save a life.

But the impact of the Hopkins case and the Duff-Campbell article was largely limited to the community of those who care for sick newborns and the ever-growing number of "bioethicists" who think and write about the moral and ethical issues involved in medical care. The third event, however, which seemingly had nothing to do with the care of newborns, proved to have a profound effect upon both the shape of the debate itself and the forum in which it was to be conducted, moving it out of the nurseries and into the nation's living rooms.

That momentous third event was the 1973 decision of the U.S. Supreme Court in the case of *Roe* v. *Wade:* the granting to women of the right to abortion on demand in the first and second trimesters of pregnancy. On its face, the legalization of abortion had little or nothing to do with the debate over the care of defective newborns. To be sure, there were those opponents of abortion who argued that legalizing abortion was the first step down the infamous "slippery slope" to infanticide and the mass murder of the weak and infirm. And those same individuals can point to the handful of publicized cases in which care was withheld from defective newborns and say, "See, we warned you." But that, of course, simply ignores the fact that infanticide of one form or another has always been with us and always will be, and the decisions that are being made today are no different from those made a decade ago except that physicians may now be even more cautious about making them because of pressure from anti-abortion activists. There were also those, like the late physician, researcher, ethicist and opponent of abortion Andre Hellegers, who said that the rationalization of abortion that most troubled him was that the fetus being aborted was defective. What does that say, Hellegers would ask, about our view of and willingness to protect the less than perfect living among us? There is really no way to reply to that kind of argument other than to say, yes, such thinking is disturbing and it suggests we should be ever vigilant in protecting the rights of the helpless individuals entrusted to our care.

In early 1982 an infant was born in Bloomington, Indiana, suffering from Down's syndrome, an esophageal atresia and a tracheoesophageal atresia as well. This last complication, a connection of the stomach with the trachea rather than the esophagus, results in bile eating away at the windpipe and often the lungs themselves. The infant's parents considered, and rejected, surgery to clear the blocked esophagus and close the connection between the stomach and the trachea. Their pediatrician concurred in the decision, which meant that the infant could not be fed and would starve to death. But another physician and some hospital personnel were deeply disturbed by the decision to withhold treatment, and the hospital insisted on taking the case to court, believing that a judge, at best, would order surgery and, at worst, would absolve the hospital and its staff from any potential criminal or civil liability should the infant die. The judge did refuse to order the potentially life-saving surgery, and the case came to the attention of both the local prosecutor and local and national right-to-life advocates. The prosecutor tried unsuccessfully to have the child declared neglected and thus in need of state protection. An appeal to a higher state court was equally unsuccessful, as was an attempt to take the case to the Supreme Court of the United States. By the time Infant Doe died, six days after his birth, the entire nation had been exposed through the media to the case of Baby Doe, whose parents were allowing it to be starved to death. While some individuals who heard of the case understood that such decisions are not uncommon, and understood why they are made, many others did not. One of those others was Ronald Reagan, President of the United States, who was said to be deeply disturbed by the thought that an infant could be allowed to starve to death.

Ronald Reagan had run in 1980 with the warm support of the nation's antiabortion movement and had promised to stop what was being termed the "slaughter of the unborn." The problem was that there was little he could do to make good on his promise. He supported Congress in its successful efforts to cut off Medicaid funds for abortions for poor women, but he was unable in his first term to do anything to bring about a reversal of the 1973 Supreme Court decision legalizing abortion. So what was to become quickly known as the Baby Doe issue gave the Reagan administration something tangible it could do for the antiabortion movement.

Spurred on by Americans United for Life, the principal legal wing of the antiabortion movement, and the American Life Lobby, which claims 130,000 members and says it is the largest pro-life, pro-family organization in the country, the White House ordered the federal Department of Health and Human Services (HHS) to inform the nation's more than 6800 hospitals and health care institutions that failing to provide nourishment or

184

necessary medical treatment to a "handicapped" newborn would place the institution in violation of Section 504 of the 1973 Rehabilitation Act. Thus, the administration was attempting to use a law passed to provide the handicapped with equal access to jobs, education and housing, a law intended to make sure that elevators were wide enough to provide access to wheelchairs, to control the way medicine was being practiced in the delivery suites and intensive care nurseries of hospitals. Not content to simply leave its warning a warning, on March 2, 1983, HHS issued its so-called Baby Doe rules, requiring that all hospital delivery suites and nurseries have posted conspicuous signs warning that "Discriminatory Failure to Feed and Care for Handicapped Infants in This Facility Is Prohibited by Federal Law." And in addition to the warning, each sign listed the toll-free telephone number of the Baby Doe hotline, an 800 number manned twenty-four hours a day by federal workers faithfully taking down the anonymous complaint of any caller, be that caller a parent, physician, nurse, nurse's aid, hospital janitor or simply someone who had "heard" about an infant being mistreated at a local hospital.

The uproar that followed was incredible. In the first place, the hotline was flooded with calls, more than 500 in the first three weeks. And the stories the callers told were appalling: March 22—ten babies were being simultaneously starved to death in a Nashville hospital; March 23—a premature infant born in a Baltimore hospital was being denied life-sustaining care; April 4—the parents and physician caring for a premature infant in Miami reportedly refused to allow necessary resuscitation; September 21—a caller complains that, in Boise, Idaho, "an abandoned premature infant with no brain tissue might be withdrawn from life support."

What did the government's special Baby Doe teams determine when they traveled to the far corners of the country to investigate these complaints? The ten infants in Nashville, being cared for in the nursery of one of America's leading neonatologists, were all receiving excellent, appropriate care. The baby in Baltimore died, having been delivered prior to the point of viability. The Miami baby the caller said was not resuscitated had died before the complaint was filed. The caller had read about the case in a newspaper but had apparently failed to note that, in addition to being premature, the infant suffered from what a summary of Baby Doe investigations termed "multiple catastrophic conditions, including complete liquefication of the brain." And the abandoned premature infant in Boise that a caller feared was being withdrawn from life support simply because it had no brain tissue? For some inexplicable reason the state "child protective services agency had obtained custody of the infant and had no plans to discontinue life support."

In addition to firing up the indignation and imagination of right-to-life tipsters around the country, the establishment of the Baby Doe rules and hotline brought the American Academy of Pediatrics, the Children's Hospital National Medical Center in Washington, and the National Association of Children's Hospitals into federal district court in Washington, D.C., seeking to have the rules overturned. Judge Gerhard Gesell struck the regulations down on a number of grounds, not the least of which was that the administration had failed to show that the regulations would in any way actually improve the medical care for those infants they were intended to protect. By June 27 HHS came back with a new set of regulations, this one at least making clear that it did not intend to compel the use of futile therapies in hopeless cases.

On October 11, 1983, before the courts could settle the question of the ultimate legality of the Baby Doe regulations, a baby girl was born in St. Charles Hospital in Port Jefferson, New York, who would come to symbolize all the dilemmas involved in the Baby Doe issue. Baby Jane Doe, as she was first publicly known, was born suffering from a constellation of birth defects, including meningomyelocele (a failure of a portion of the neural tube to form properly, thus exposing an area of spinal cord in her lower back), a malformed left foot, paralysis of the legs, anal incontinence, mild hydrocephalus, microcephaly (an abnormally small head, and thus an abnormally small brain, for her size) and certain facial characteristics indicative of retardation.

Initially unaware of any problem other than the meningomyelocele, the parents authorized their daughter's transfer to University Hospital at Stony Brook, a state teaching hospital. It is unlikely we will ever really know who told what to whom during those first few days at Stony Brook, but after initially signing an authorization for anesthesia for surgery, the parents refused to authorize the surgery necessary to close the opening in their daughter's back. As he later testified in court, neurologist George Newman, who examined the infant, believed that "on the basis of the combinations of the malformations that are present in this child she is not likely to ever achieve any meaningful interactions with her environment, nor ever to achieve any interpersonal relationships that we consider human, and that she is capable of experiencing pain." Newman further testified that because he believed the infant had "only limited ability to experience comfort, and primarily an ability to experience pain, to perform this surgery would increase the total pain that the child would experience. There are complications of the [meningomyelocele], including urinary tract infections, skin infections, edema of the legs, and numerous other conditions, all of which would produce pain and none of which might be detectable before they produce pain in the child." Not surprisingly, the parents refused to authorize what they were told would be life-extending surgery to close the spinal defect. According to a social worker's note in the early medical record, the baby's father had somehow been led to believe she would die within twenty-four hours without surgery and was quite upset emotionally when she didn't.

It would have been difficult enough for the parents, physicians and nurses caring for this Baby Doe had they simply had to live with the decision that had been made and care for the infant. Medical personnel knew full well that infants with spina bifida, as the combination of the open spine and hydrocephalus is known, vary enormously in their outcome. With surgery to close the spine and a shunt to drain the fluid buildup in the skull, many of these children do quite well. They usually suffer from paralysis of the legs and are unable to control their bladders, but a good number learn to walk with braces and some have normal intelligence. At the other end of the spectrum are children such as neurologist Newman described in court, children who are crippled, profoundly retarded and lead existences of painful desperation. But those caring for Baby Jane Doe had more to worry about than whether they made the right choice for her: On Saturday, October 15, just four days after the infant's birth, New York Supreme Court Justice Frank DeLuca, Vermont attorney and zealous right-to-life advocate Lawrence Washburn, an assistant Suffolk County district attorney and another private attorney appeared at University Hospital for a "brief, off-the-record, judicial inquiry" into the case of Baby Jane Doe. As soon as he managed to contact the attorney for the university, the administrator on duty at the hospital sent the four men packing, politely telling them to file a formal complaint if they had anything to discuss. While there was never any public discussion of how the case came to Washburn's, and thus the court's, attention, university officials have said they assume that someone at St. Charles Hospital heard that surgery was not being performed at Stony Brook and notified a local antiabortion group that in turn contacted Washburn.

The following day Washburn formally asked the state supreme court, the lower court in New York, to order that the baby remain at Stony Brook, to appoint a temporary guardian to

188

authorize surgery and to order a neurosurgeon to perform the surgery. Following two days of hearings, at which the testimony made it quite clear that, while there might be differences of medical opinion as to whether or not surgery should be performed, the parents' choice of nontreatment was well within normal bounds, the judge hearing the case found for Washburn, appointing a guardian and ordering surgery. Just one day later, a five-judge panel of the supreme court's Appellate Division reversed the ruling. "This is not a case where an infant is being deprived of medical treatment to achieve a quick and supposedly merciful death," the appeals court found. "Rather it is a situation where the parents have chosen one course of appropriate medical treatment over another. These concededly concerned and loving parents made an informed, intelligent and reasonable determination based upon and supported by responsible medical authority."

And that should have been the end of the case of Baby Jane Doe. But it wasn't. Instead, on October 23 a federal Baby Doe investigator arrived on Long Island to review the records in the case. However, rather than comply with the government's demand that the records be produced, state officials refused, and the investigator returned to Washington empty-handed. Two days later the local attorney who was originally appointed Baby Doe's temporary guardian appealed the decision of the lower appeals court to the New York Court of Appeals, the state's highest court. Thus, there were two parallel, yet quite separate, legal battles being waged over Baby Doe, one to "save" her with surgery her parents did not want for her and one to compel the hospital to allow the federal government to examine her records to determine if her civil rights were being violated.

The two fights dragged on for months, and the parents and the hospital were upheld by the courts at every stage. New York state's highest court held that the case did not belong in the courts in the first place because the legislature had intended that such issues be dealt with by state agencies utilizing the child protection statutes. To allow an outsider like Washburn to bring such cases into court, the high court found, would ". . . catapult him into the very heart of the family circle, there to challenge the most private and precious responsibility vested in parents for the care and nurture of their children." The court-appointed guardian attempted to take the case to the U.S. Supreme Court but was refused a hearing, without comment. Washburn then filed a class-action suit in U.S. District Court on behalf of all infants like Jane Doe, claiming that they were being denied their civil rights, and asked that a new temporary guardian be appointed for the infant. Not only did the court not rule in Washburn's favor, but Judge Roger J. Miner went so far as to fine Washburn for violating that portion of the federal Rules of Civil Procedure that forbids bringing a case to "harass or to cause unnecessary delay or needlessly increase the cost of litigation." The Vermont attorney appealed the ruling, but then withdrew the appeal and withdrew from the case as part of an agreement that resulted in the court's action against him being dropped.

On the civil rights front, the Justice Department lost at every turn. A three-judge panel of the U.S. District Court ruled two to one on February 3, 1984, that "Congress never contemplated that section 504 of the Rehabilitation Act would apply to treatment decisions involving defective newborn infants," either when the act was first passed in 1973 or when it was amended in 1984. In addition, the court held that "until Congress has spoken, it would be an unwarranted exercise of judicial power to approve the type of investigation that has precipitated this lawsuit." The government was then denied a rehearing before the entire court, and eventually decided against appealing to the U.S. Court of Appeals. The Justice Department did, however, appeal the case of the Baby Doe regulations all the way to the Supreme

Court, which agreed in June 1985 to hear the case the following term.

On October 9, 1984, President Ronald Reagan signed the Child Abuse Amendments of 1984. This Baby Doe law, which represents a compromise between such diverse groups as the American Academy of Pediatrics and national right-to-life organizations, forbids the withholding of nourishment or "medically indicated treatment" unless an infant is comatose, the treatment would only prolong dying, or the treatment would be "futile in terms of the survival of the infant." In other words, physicians are legally forbidden to include quality-of-life considerations when treating deformed or severely retarded newborns. And yet another set of Baby Doe rules, albeit without a hotline, was in effect at the end of 1985.

But what of Baby Jane Doe, the human being who, along with her parents and physicians, was the seemingly forgotten central figure in this Kafkaesque drama? Each twist in the infant's case left the initial medical assessment, and the parents' resolve, more open to question. In the first place, while the parents had decided not to authorize the closing of the spinal opening, which would drastically reduce the chances of life-threatening infections, and refused to authorize the insertion of a shunt to drain fluid from the skull and reduce the chances of further brain damage, they did authorize the use of antibiotics to fight the infections the baby quickly developed. Additionally, on November 6, 1983, about a week after they won the right to withhold treatment from the infant, the parents authorized the insertion of not one but two tubes to allow the direct insertion of antibiotics into the baby's skull to fight an infection. The effect of the tubes was to drain the same fluid the shunt would have been draining. The parents visited their infant, whom they had named Keri-Lynn, every day over the months she was in the newborn intensive care unit of University Hospital, obviously becoming more and more

191

attached to her. Finally, when she was about five months old, they authorized the insertion of the shunt whose insertion outsiders had attempted to compel five months earlier.

One of the ironies in the case is that the original medical testimony looks less and less accurate as time passes. By six months, the infant who would never be responsive was cooing and carrying on with obvious pleasure at bath time. By a year she was reportedly functioning on about a six-month level, responding to her parents, grasping at objects, enjoying toys. Would she ever progress beyond that level? That is another question. But an even more important question is, would she progress further had her spinal defect been closed and a shunt been inserted shortly after birth? The obvious answer to that question would seem to be yes. In matters such as this, however, every answer seems to pose a question, which in this case is: Does the fact that she might have done better had surgery been performed mean that surgery should have been performed?

A strong argument can be made that this was the "wrong" Baby Doe to be the central figure in a precedent-setting case. A case involving an infant like Cara Lynn Bailey, who possesses none of the attributes and abilities we equate with personhood and humanity, would have made the issues far clearer, the lines far easier to draw. But isn't the very point of the Baby Doe question that there are no easy answers? Every case comes with not one Hobson's choice but an entire set. Each case leaves another set of parents wondering if they made the right choices, whether they withheld medical treatment—or authorized it. Ultimately, the entire crushing weight of such life-and-death decision making falls on two persons, the mother and father of the infant involved. Once the baby either dies or goes home, the case ends for the physicians and nurses involved. They may think about it once in a while, they may even have a nightmare or two, but they do not live with the decision on a daily basis. They do not have to live with knowing that they decided that *their* child would be better off dead. Or, alternately, they do not have to care for a severely handicapped child for the rest of their lives. The physicians and nurses are not the ones who have to fight with the state and federal bureaucracies for every penny of the often inadequate aid the parents of such an infant receive. If the child is eventually institutionalized, the physicians and nurses do not have to go to the institution, to be bowled over by the stench of urine and disinfectant, to see a wholly inadequate number of attendants attempting to care for the castoffs of society. And, of . course, the right-to-life advocates who would save every infant, no matter how badly deformed or hopelessly retarded, are, in the vast majority of cases, nowhere to be seen except on picket lines and in court. As Marty Bailey, who knows of what she speaks, asked, "Where are they? They step into a life, do their thing and good-bye. . . . These people save a life, clap their hands after it's done and then they turn away."

There have always been mechanisms for protecting the helpless and making sure that the traditional medical decision-making process is not abused. Perhaps decisions involving the care of hopelessly ill and defective newborns should be left to those traditional processes, to parents and physicians who do the best they can under difficult circumstances. Until such time as society is willing to pay the bill for truly humane institutions or twenty-four-hour home care for all such infants, to offer families alternatives other than death or living death, shouldn't these decisions be left to those who will have to live with them?

VI.
ORGAN REPLACEMENT

CHAPTER 11

Philip Koerner's
Second Heart

Philip Koerner was a simple man with simple tastes. He was a skilled blue-collar worker whose idea of a good time was to take his wife of thirty-four years, Catherine, out to dinner or to the local bowling alley, or to go on a trip to the beach with his family. In 1963 he bought a piece of the traditional American dream—a little house in the suburbs—and moved his wife and three young children from their overcrowded apartment in Queens to Long Island. Seven years and another child later, Phil and Cathy moved to a neat, modest ranch house on a block of similar houses in Wantagh, also on Long Island. Both moves meant that Phil had to put up with long hours of commuting by train to his paper cutter's job on the night shift in a Manhattan book bindery, but he was more than willing to take the stress and strains. Someday, he liked to tell Cathy, he would retire and start a hot dog stand, working a few hours a day and taking it easy the rest of the time. But until then, he would be satisfied with the life he had made, and his income of about $30,000 a year in 1978.

The devastating physical, emotional and financial impact of major illness was not something Phil Koerner had ever had to contemplate, much less worry about. He had always been in good health, and he had been protected by his union's health insurance plan for almost thirty years.

Then, in the early hours of one Saturday morning in 1978, Phil Koerner started to have chest pains at work. "He was going to take my youngest son and seven of his buddies to an Islander game that Saturday evening," Cathy recalled, seven difficult years later. "He met me in Brooklyn to bring my mother out to recover from a heart condition. He had some chest pains, but we just thought it was some indigestion, we never gave a heart attack a thought. He drove home here and he went downstairs to lie down for a few hours, and unbeknownst to me it was getting worse and worse, the chest pains. He came up and said, 'I don't know if I'm going to make it to the game tonight; I don't feel too well.' He made it to the bathroom. I never open the bathroom door on him, never. But I just had a feeling, so I looked in and he was totally gray. I called an ambulance and they took him to the local hospital. They said it was very, very severe. They didn't know if he'd survive it. He was in the hospital forty-five days. Surgery wasn't for him. It was the heart muscle itself. At that time they were into bypasses and all that, but it wasn't for him."

Phil "wasn't told to quit," Cathy said, "but he was out of work for about a year. He was going to a center for heart patients to build himself up. My husband loved his work, and of course we liked the money," she said. Cathy and Phil did not even know how much Phil's forty-five days of hospitalization and year of rehabilitation cost. They had to pay a few thousand dollars in co-payments, but the great bulk of the charges were paid directly by the union's Blue Cross and major medical plans.

When Phil finally went back to work, Cathy said. "He had cut out all the overtime and was just grateful to be back working. Little by little he'd put in an hour of overtime here and an hour there. We'd argue about it. He stopped, but it got to the point where he had another heart attack. I think the commuting had a lot to do with it. The Long Island Railroad. The train would be late and he'd get so aggravated with them: 'You pay a fortune for your ticket and look what you get!' "

Like the first attack, the second also began early on a Saturday morning, about a year after Phil had resumed working. "He had started with the pains at work and he knew what was coming," Cathy said, "so he came home because he was so afraid of being stuck in a hospital in the city. He came right home to me and I took him to the hospital."

Phil spent thirty days in the hospital following the second attack, and, for the second time, the physicians told Cathy that "they couldn't understand how he was surviving. People with less damage than he had had died. After about six months he went back to work and he worked about three months and he came home one day and he said, 'I know I can't do it anymore.' The fellas at work would try to help him and such, with things he couldn't do, but he just felt that he was such a burden on everybody and really felt like, I guess, that his manhood was taken away from him. In fact," Cathy recalled, "he didn't even tell the men that he was retiring. The last night he was there the big bosses came in, they're not usually there at night. And they put on a big spread for him and everybody was totally shocked—his co-workers—because nobody knew he was going to retire. And he left work that night around four in the morning and around eight in the morning I said, 'That son of a gun is working overtime his last night at work, I'm going to really murder him! I can't stand it!' I called the place and they said, 'Phil left at four in the morning.' Well, for sure I had him laying dead, mugged someplace on the subways. But he was riding the subways all night, crying, the whole night, because he had to leave his job. He just loved it." She began to cry. "He didn't get home till about twelve-thirty that afternoon."

When forty-nine-year-old Phil Koerner retired in 1981, after

199

twenty-eight years of bindery work, he qualified for a union pension of $470 a month. He also qualified for a Social Security disability benefit of about $640, giving him an income of about $1100 a month. "I'd been working part-time, as a medical secretary, for the past fifteen years, but I started working full-time when he got sick and tried to take up the slack," Cathy said.

Because of the extent of Phil's disability, "There wasn't much of anything he could do. He cooked for me—he became a gourmet cook. What a cook! He'd do laundry. Little things that he could do for me to try to help out. We're from the old times," Cathy explained, "where a man felt that he should take care of the woman and in a way I did too. A woman likes to feel taken care of, I guess. The adjustment was hard at first. It was *my* kitchen. But little by little I figured, why be a jerk—if he wants to cook, let him cook. I'd come home to a big mess, but I'd do anything to have that mess again." Again, she had to pause to wipe away tears.

The adjustment to forced retirement was even harder for Phil. "He couldn't even talk to the fellas at work because he'd cry for days after. Phil was a foreman, and the one fella who got his job made $65,000 last year. He'd say, 'Hey, Phil, look what I made!' and that used to just kill him. . . ." The physical adjustment to infirmity was no easier than the psychological adjustment. "Spring and summer he always used to seem to thrive. Come fall and winter, he'd seem to deteriorate. In the spring and summer he was seen once a month [by his doctor], but in the winter it would be at least twice a month. And then the depression would set in because he couldn't go out," Cathy said.

The medical bills were initially paid by Phil's union insurance plan, but then, two and one-half years after he began receiving Social Security, he qualified for Medicare. At that point, Cathy recalled, the union coverage "was cut back drastically. And, as you know, Medicare, in what they'll allow, has been drastically cut back too. I really don't know what the older people do," Cathy said, bitter about what she saw as the lack of support from a system she and millions of other Americans have always assumed would be there when they needed it. "And my husband really should have had somebody here to take care of him," she continued, "but I hadda go to work. If I had stayed home and gone on welfare, we would have had an aide. But because we wouldn't go on welfare, we, I, have all these bills and my husband had to be alone. I don't know how my boss put up with it all those years. I'd get at least five phone calls a day from Phil, or I'd be calling home to check up on him. It's a terrible strain on you, a big worry. If the phone didn't answer in five rings you'd worry."

Meanwhile, Phil Koerner's health continued to deteriorate. By the time he had been retired two years he had had two more heart attacks. Through a friend, Cathy heard about Deborah Heart and Lung Hospital in Browns Mills, New Jersey, and physicians there managed to adjust Phil's many medications to the point where he at least stabilized for a while. But by the winter of 1984–85, he reached the point where he had to make weekly trips to the doctor. And "he didn't seem to pick up as he had been by the spring. One day the doctor had him in one of the examining rooms and he came out and he said, 'How's he doing at home?' I said, 'I'm really worried because it seems to be getting very bad.' This was, I guess, the end of April. He said, 'It's not going to get any better, Cathy. The only thing that may help is a transplant.' Well, you could a picked me up off the floor! He told me to feel Phil out. When we got home I said, 'Oh God, I just wish they could give you a transplant!' He said, 'What are you, crazy? Are you nuts?' I said, 'No, I think it could help you.'"

The next week, during Phil's weekly checkup at the local hospital, another physician was brought in to examine him, and that specialist, too, said he needed a transplant if he was to have a chance at surviving more than about six months. But as Cathy remembered it a few months later, "His words to me were, 'He's fifty-five years old, the criteria in New York is forty-five, and besides, where would you get $250,000?' I just looked at him. I didn't know what to say. Well, it got to the point where he [Phil] couldn't eat, he couldn't eat a morsel of food. One night we managed to get him out to the dinner table and he took one bite and he was vomiting all over the table. That night I prayed. I said, 'Give me some kind of an answer.' You just can't watch your husband die like that without doing something. The next morning Deborah Hospital came to mind. In the meantime I had mentioned transplant to him again. I mentioned Deborah Hospital and he said, 'Take me there, whatever they say I will do. . . .' "

May 6, 1985, Philip Koerner entered Deborah Heart and Lung for what was supposed to be a three-day examination. His condition was so bad, however, that "They wanted at that time to fly him down by helicopter to [the Milton S.] Hershey Medical Center," in Hershey, Pennsylvania, to be evaluated for a heart transplant. "But he wanted to come home," Cathy said. "I guess he felt he was coming home one last time. They wanted to send him home in an ambulance. He said, 'I'll drive home with my wife.'

"That Sunday, the twelfth, was Mother's Day," Cathy continued. "The thirteenth was my birthday. So we celebrated my birthday on Sunday," and on Monday, the day Catherine Koerner turned fifty, she drove her husband the five hours to the Hershey Medical Center, where he insisted on walking in under his own power, rather than be admitted in a wheelchair. As Cathy recalled, "He said, 'If I walk in that hospital, I'll walk out.' Which he did."

Cathy said that after Phil was assessed she was told that he was a candidate for a heart transplant because, even though he was over fifty-five, his other organs were still in excellent condition, except for his lungs, which had suffered some damage because of the heart condition. But at that point it looked as though he could lead a relatively normal life if he survived the transplant. The odds on survival, she was told, were 80 percent the first year and 50-50 for each succeeding year. "They told us that Medicare would not pay for the transplant," Cathy said. "I was shocked. I said, 'Well, we have health insurance,' But because Medicare doesn't approve transplants, the union plan won't pay for it either. They told us up-front that it was $100,000, that's just the hospital, excluding the doctor. The surgeon said, 'Your husband needs the operation, without it he's not going to live. I will do it, and afterwards we'll discuss it [the money].' He said, 'I don't want you to even worry about that.' He was wonderful. They kept Phil there one week. Normally what they do is send them home with a beeper to wait for a heart. But his condition was so bad they said he'd never make it home."

On Tuesday, May 22, a twenty-year-old Pennsylvania man died in a motorcycle accident and gave Philip Koerner at fifty-five a second life. The transplant operation went smoothly, and before long Cathy Koerner was worrying more about how she would ever be able to pay the more than $100,000 hospital bill—exclusive of any physicians' charges—than she was about whether Phil would survive. "You always think you're going to be one of the lucky ones. You think that if he made it through that surgery, he'd make it," she said. Realizing that the bill was already astronomical, and realizing that it did not include hundreds of dollars a month for medications, or the weekly, and later monthly, $3000 checkups Phil would need, Cathy told officials at Hershey that she would sell the family home to pay the bills. "But they said, 'No, where can you go?' They knew approximately how much it cost to live up here. It was amazing. They said it would be traumatic for Phil not to go home to his own home. Those people down there were so wonderful. They were always so pleasant. They couldn't do enough for you. They said that what people usually do in situations like this is they start a fund."

So that is what Cathy did. Although the hospital never said it would accept what was raised by the fund as full payment, she established a special bank account and made public appeals for help. *Newsday* ran several stories about her husband's plight. Neighbors held "the biggest garage sale on Long Island" and raised about $2000. The insurance company that employed one of her daughters raffled off a gold watch and cleared about $11,000. All together, friends and strangers paid about $18,000 toward Phil Koerner's transplant. But "It's a very, very demeaning thing. It's very heartwarming. Everybody who sent us a check sent us a warm little note. You just don't realize that people really do care. We'd sit here some nights," she said, sitting in her comfortably furnished living room, "just reading over the notes and the letters. But it was still demeaning. We'd never taken charity before."

During June and early July everything went well for Phil. "He could breathe again for the first time in years. And I didn't know he'd been in pain, but he told me, 'For the first time in seven years I don't have pain in my chest,' " Cathy recalled. "We went to the movies, which we hadn't in I can't tell you how long. We went out to dinner a couple of times. We'd always go to a restaurant when it wasn't too crowded, because he had to go in with his mask on [in order to avoid infection] and then we'd get situated where there weren't too many people." During one of Phil's trips to Hershey for a weekly examination and biopsy of the new heart to monitor rejection, he had fresh pineapple for dessert in the motel restaurant and "his mouth started to burn. He got sores all over his mouth and we were frightened that they'd keep him there. It was such a traumatic thing. When he told the [transplant program] coordinator, very sheepishly, about it, she said, 'Don't worry about that! We have a medicine for that! There isn't anything you can get now, Phil, that we don't have a medicine for.' Whewwww! What a relief."

But all that medication was far from benign. By mid-July Phil was suffering from excruciating pain in his back. Cathy called Hershey "and they said take him to an orthopedist here, so I work for an orthopedist and he took X rays" and discovered that Phil had fractured several vertebrae weakened by the cylosporine he was taking to prevent rejection of his new heart. "We called the hospital and they said follow the orders of the orthopedist, and we did," Cathy recalled. The orthopedist "said Phil had to get up and walk around because they're afraid of pneumonia setting in. Then his leg started to swell, he started retaining some water in the legs. And I called them on that, and at that point he had almost reached his monthly checkup. This was going into the third week in July and they put him on a water pill. They put him on it on a Friday and by Saturday he was swollen up to his knees and he could hardly walk and I was so terrified that he was going to get pneumonia." Family members and friends got Phil out of bed and helped him spend part of the day walking around the backyard. Saturday night, Cathy said, Phil began coughing in his sleep. "That Sunday morning, to get him up out of the bed was a horror story. He had to literally crawl out and I had to lift him up. Even though he was only one hundred and twenty-five pounds it was really hard. He said, 'Honey, if I cough tonight'— he didn't know he'd been coughing—'then we'll talk about going down earlier.' He just knew something was going on and he was frightened. That night he went to bed and he was coughing the whole night in his sleep, he didn't even know he was coughing. He was bringing up bile, I was wiping it from his mouth the whole night. In the morning, at seven, I called the doctor here and I said, 'He won't listen to me, he won't go back there. Please come over and check him out.' He said, 'Cathy, I can come over, but what good is it? I can't do anything. You've got to get him back there.' So he spoke to my husband on the phone and my husband said, 'Okay, I'll go back.' I called his best friend, Harold, and we got him down to Hershey. It was five hours of torture for him with his back, he was in such agony."

Cathy continued: "So we got him down there and the doctor looked at his legs and right away they started giving him intravenous with diuretics in it. The doctor said, 'Phil, what am I going to do with you? Now you're going to make me work for your money.' I knew it was serious, but he tried to make light of it. And then the next day Phil's legs were almost back to normal already, and I was really very encouraged. And a lung man came in, and the lung man said, 'He has tuberculosis.' I said, 'WHAT!?' I said, 'Where could he get that from?' He said, 'It's in the air, but not to worry, within ten days they'll have him cured of that.' We all had to go for patch tests, but they were negative. Wednesday I had to leave him. The doctor said, 'It's going to take him months, if he survives.' I said. 'Oh, he'll survive. The legs are already down and the TB's only going to take ten days. He'll survive. The legs are already down.' And he said, 'Cathy, Phil's a very, very sick man.' I said, 'I know that, but he's been sicker. Are you giving up on him?' He said, 'No, no, of course not.' 'Well, don't expect me to,' I told him.

"I drove home and all the way back I had a funny feeling. I said to this friend, Harold, I said, 'If I turn the block and I see my children's cars there I'll know something's wrong.' But there were no cars by the house. So I came in very light-hearted." But she found her daughter waiting for her with news that the hospital had called: Phil had taken a turn for the worse and was on a respirator. Cathy turned around and headed back for Hershey, accompanied by her children.

"Friday morning the doctor said, 'If he survives, I told you before, it's going to take months. So go home, do what you have to do and come down on weekends.' I was all set to go, in fact we put my one daughter on a plane to go home. She got off the plane in New York and an hour later she was on the plane coming back, because she just had a strong feeling about it. She said she had to be there with me. At the last minute, I was coming home in the car with my other daughter and my two sons. I said, 'I'm not going. I just can't go.' So my daughter stayed with me and my other daughter came back with her fiancé."

Cathy stayed in the intensive care unit with Phil until about 10 P.M. on Friday, and then went back to her motel room to sleep. Saturday morning, August 10, Cathy "called them from the motel and I said, 'How was his night?' And the nurse said, 'He had a very hard night.' I said, 'I'll be over in a few minutes,' and she said, 'Yes, come as soon as you can.' "

Thirty minutes later, Cathy was at her husband's bedside. "You know all those machines, the whole room was machines. They had him on a respirator, and I used to sing a couple songs to him . . ." She paused, choking back tears, and then regained her composure and continued, ". . . and he didn't respond anymore to them. I said to the nurse, 'Geez, what are all those numbers, explain them to me.' She said, 'Well, the top number's his heartbeat.' It was 127. I said, 'Well that's his lucky number, it's my son's birthday, 12/7. Once in a while he'd play that number. He never won on it, but he'd play that number once in a while,' and she just gave a smirk. I said, 'What's that other number?' She said, 'That's his blood pressure.' I said, 'Gee, that's kind of low, isn't it, but then he does run low blood pressure.' She said, 'That's very low.' I said, 'How much lower can it get?' She said, 'Very low, until there's none.' I said, 'You don't expect that, do you?' She said. 'Yes, I do.' And by ten o'clock he was gone."

Philip Koerner died of heart failure eighty days after getting his new heart. His system had been overwhelmed by a fungal infection that got a foothold because his immune system was so effectively suppressed by the drugs intended to prevent rejection of the transplanted heart. Thus, he died of an iatrogenic disease, a disease caused by the very medical care designed to save his life. And he died leaving his widow well over $125,000 in medical bills she cannot conceivably pay on her $259-a-week take-home pay as a medical secretary.

A month after Phil's death Cathy still had not seen a bill for his final stay in the hospital. "I'm afraid I may need a transplant when I see it," she said, with a false laugh, "and Medicare doesn't pay anything on that last visit either because it all revolves around the heart transplant." Cathy explained that she had "made an agreement with them [Hershey] that I would send them $2000 a month, when the fund started to grow. At first I said, 'I'll send whatever I get.' They said, 'No, send us $2000 per month, and this way there'll always be some money in the fund and it will earn some interest and you can always keep adding to the fund.' " But with her husband dead, and little prospect of increasing the fund, Cathy said she didn't know what to do. She hadn't called Hershey to discuss the problem, either. "I'm afraid," she said softly. "I'm actually afraid. My husband and I had kidded that they couldn't repossess the heart. But I don't know what to do." (Officials at Hershey later said they would collect whatever was in the fund, and whatever insurance would pay, but said they would not pursue the matter further.)

"It was over too fast for us," Cathy said, thinking about the transplant experience. "But Sunday mornings here are a big time. My kids are all here and we have breakfast together. This one beautiful Sunday morning Phil had been home about two weeks and he just started crying out in the back. He said, 'If I die tomorrow, I'll die a happy man.' He could breathe again. He could eat. He could walk. He could enjoy people. My husband wasn't the type of man who would go and sit in somebody's house on his own. We'd go visit our friends, but to just go into somebody else's house, a neighbor's, just to knock on the door to visit them, he never in his life had done that. But this one day I'm looking for him and he had gone to visit two neighbors who were dying of cancer. He had gone over there to visit them to encourage them to ask the Lord for a miracle. He'd gotten a miracle and they could too. And when he died, both those women said, 'Now we'll never get our miracle.'. . . I said, 'Phil did get his miracle. We were the stupid ones. We didn't ask for ten years or twenty years.

"It was a very traumatic thing. The whole family has suffered. But we wouldn't trade one minute because there were a lot of memories too, there was a lot of happiness. When you see them get out of bed for the first time, see them take their first steps. And when they start eating: I thought I was going to have to put a lock on the fridge because this man was eating everything in sight. That was such a happy sight. I think God gives you a chance and you have to take it. Why did he give these people all this knowledge if he didn't want you to try?

"I think that people who need [financial] help should get it. I am very resentful. How much did it cost for the President's last surgery and who paid for that?" she asked sarcastically. "I know it cost a hell of a lot more than my husband's surgery with all that security. And we give all this money away to other countries. Why should somebody who works all his life, and then I went out to work, have to go through this? If we'd gone on welfare he could have had everything paid for, but you don't want welfare. My husband was a proud man."

Are the chances of a good outcome oversold? she was asked.

"I knew the odds, but I felt that if he survived that surgery. . . ." She paused, and then continued, "They take a heart out and they hold it in their hand. It's such a traumatic, dramatic thing. It's unreal. These people are fighting to save lives. You just hope that someday it will really help. It's helping people now. You never give up. I still can't believe that he's gone. In fact, they had told my husband that his condition was so bad that if it got to a point where if they had to sustain life would be have gone on the machine [the Jarvik-7 artificial heart, which Hershey has approval to use as a temporary measure for patients awaiting a human heart]? At first he said no. But then, you want to live so bad that he said he would do it."

CHAPTER 12

Transplanting Life

It is difficult, if not impossible, to argue with someone like Catherine Koerner when she says that ". . . people who need [financial] help should get it. . . . Why should somebody who works all his life . . . have to go through this? If we'd gone on welfare he could have had everything paid for, but you don't want welfare." After all, isn't one of the motivations for a life of hard work the idea that we are preparing ourselves for the proverbial rainy day? Clearly, no average individual can prepare for the kind of financial hurricane unleashed by the need for a heart transplant, but we assume that when such a storm comes, the government we have supported with a lifetime of ever-increasing tax payments will provide us with the care we ourselves cannot afford.

At this point, there is no clear federal government policy on the financing of organ transplants. This is not to say there are not policies, for there are. But they are neither clear nor singular. For instance, Medicare, the federally funded health insurance plan for the aged and disabled, classifies heart, heart-lung and liver transplants for adults as experimental procedures, and thus pays neither for the transplant operation nor for the expensive aftercare. Medicare will, however, pay for some of these transplants for children—but more about that later. Medicaid, the joint state-federal health insurance program for the indigent, does pay for such transplants—in some states. Thus, Catherine Koerner was correct when she bitterly noted that had she and her husband been willing to go on welfare, their medical bills would have been paid.

To make the matter of government funding even more confusing, at the same time Medicare refuses to pay for any costs related to heart transplantation, the program pays virtually all the expenses related to kidney transplantation and its lifetime of aftercare. When we consider organ tranplantation on a case-by-case basis and know the individuals involved as individuals, it is logical to conclude that the government's handling of kidney transplantation and dialysis (the use of the artificial kidney) should set the pattern for the way in which we treat those needing other types of organ transplants. Before we act on that conclusion, however, there are a number of factors to consider.

First, compared with other major organ transplants, a kidney transplant is cheap at $25,000 to $30,000. Second, the one-year survival rate for patients who receive a kidney from a living, related donor is about 96 percent, while those who receive cadaver kidneys have about a 90-percent survival rate. Because of the use of extremely expensive antirejection drugs, such as cylosporine—which may cost the patient about $8000 per year—the five-year organ survival rate is now around 80 percent. The reason organ and patient mortality rates can be considered separately in the case of kidney transplants is that patients whose transplanted organs fail can be placed on dialysis to await a new organ. Third, and perhaps most important, the cost of keeping a person alive with dialysis in two years outstrips the cost of a transplant, so a successful transplant unquestionably represents a savings to the individual and society. But it is impossible to consider the public funding of kidney transplants without also examining the financing of the dialysis program, so let's briefly consider the history of government involvement in organ substitution, the use of artificial organs and the transplantation of both natural and artificial organs.

Unlike the victims of other types of organ failure, persons suffering from end-stage renal disease (ESRD)—kidney failure—can physically lead relatively normal lives if they are provided with artificial dialysis, the cleansing of the blood several times a week with a mechanical kidney. Some patients do remarkably well on dialysis: They master the machine, making it an adjunct to their lives, a minor annoyance and even, in some cases, a mechanical friend. They live full, rich lives, pursuing careers, supporting and caring for families, contributing to the lives of their friends and communities. The majority, however, lead what can best be described as "lives of quiet desperation," dependent psychologically, as well as physically, on the machine that sustains their lives. They do not work. They are not involved in the world around them. And they opt out of that world at an astounding rate: According to one study, the suicide rate among dialysis patients is four hundred times the national average.

Whether dialysis treatments free an individual or become a kind of psychological and physical torture, they do not come cheap. And when the treatment was first perfected in the early 1960s by Dr. Belding H. Scribner at the University of Washington in Seattle, the treatment was neither cheap nor widely available. From 1962, when *Life* magazine ran a major article on Scribner's work, to 1972, when the federal ESRD program was established, there were a number of articles in both lay and professional publications about the awful dilemma facing those who controlled access to the few dialysis programs around the country. In order to be one of the lucky patients allowed in the Seattle program, one had to first be screened by a medical committee

213

and then win the approval of an anonymous "God Committee," which weighed the relative value to society of the individuals competing for the few available openings in the dialysis programs. As Professor Richard A. Rettig, chairman of the Department of Social Sciences at the Illinois Institute of Technology, noted in a 1982 article entitled "The Federal Government and Social Planning for End-Stage Renal Disease: Past, Present, and Future," the federal government spent a decade ducking the question of what to do about establishing an ESRD program. For instance, when in August 1963 the *Wall Street Journal* ran an article on the hard choices facing those controlling access to the dialysis programs, "White House staff asked HEW for background on the availability or scarcity of life-saving artificial kidney machines," Rettig wrote. "HEW responded that no funds were earmarked for renal disease, but did enumerate the possible sources of support. No further action occurred," noted Rettig, who studied the ESRD program for more than a decade.

Congress, however, did not totally ignore the problem. In fact, throughout the 1960s and into the early 1970s more than one hundred pieces of legislation concerning the problem were introduced. But not one of them even received a hearing. Then, in October 1972, the late Senator Vance Hartke (D-Ind.) took the Senate floor and in a matter of minutes convinced his colleagues to include in the Medicare program all persons with end-stage renal disease, regardless of their age or ability to pay for treatment. Hartke had a compelling argument: For those with failed kidneys, the only thing standing between life and death was money. There was no other disease or disease process where this line of demarcation was—or is—so clear. Dialysis was scarce and horrifically expensive, and the very idea of God committees was un-American. Never before, or since, for that matter, has a single disease category been included in the Social Security/Medicare program with no consideration of the age of the patient. But

214

Hartke was persuasive, and Section 2991 was included in the Social Security Amendments of 1972. From then on, any patient with failing kidneys, whether six months old with a full life ahead or age ninety-five with intractable cancer and heart disease, was entitled to government-funded dialysis and any number of transplants that might be needed, should the matching organs be found. It was predicted the program would cost $250 million a year by its fourth year, but the Senate approved Section 2991, considering the price an acceptable one to pay to save the lives of tens of thousands of kidney disease patients each year. The wooden horse had entered the city.

Within months of the passage of Section 2991, it became apparent that $500 million was a more accurate projection of the program's fourth-year cost, and it would not be long before the costs topped the $1-billion mark. Because the program keeps patients alive at all stages of life, and because transplantation is limited by both the gross availability of organs and the necessity to tissue-match the recipient and the donor organ as closely as possible, the numbers of persons being maintained by dialysis is ever-increasing. In 1980 there were 52,364 patients on dialysis, and by 1983 that number had risen to 71,987, with 6,112 receiving transplants that year. In less than a decade a program that was originally to maintain the lives of about 10,000 patients had grown to care for more than 73,000—at a cost to the federal government of more than $2 billion a year. It is estimated that unless the number of patients on dialysis can be greatly reduced by providing transplants or the cost of dialysis can be greatly reduced—and neither prospect appears particularly bright—by the turn of the decade we will be paying some $600,000 per patient for the fifteen years of treatment the average dialysis patient receives before dying. This might seem a cheap price to pay were all the patients infants, or even young adults, who would then have relatively full lives ahead of them. But such is not the case.

215

Many of the patients are elderly individuals suffering from one or more chronic or acute conditions, and many of the younger individuals do not end up living anything that can be even charitably called a full life. As George Annas, Utley Professor of Health Law at Boston University School of Medicine and a noted authority on patients' rights, puts it, "Economically and in terms of providing quality care, the program has been a disaster, since the incentives to most nephrologists [kidney specialists] are to keep patients on dialysis (that is the only way they make money). In fact, most people think that instead of transplanting one-third of the patients we have fewer than ten percent on waiting lists for organs."

All of this, of course, begs the question: Can we, faced with a $200-billion deficit, spend almost $2 billion a year providing a handful of patients with a therapy that provides a quality of life that is questionable? Can we rationalize making this kind of expenditure at a time when we are cutting childhood immunization programs and basic Medicare reimbursement? Granted, society has a moral obligation to those individuals who are already in the ESRD program. But is it not time to put a cap of some kind on the program for future years and future patients? Is it not time to say that, at some certain future date, we will deal with dialysis as the British do, placing an age limit on those considered for the treatment? Or should we reclassify dialysis as an acute-care technology, only to be used for a fixed period of time to give a patient a chance to undergo a transplant?

And should Medicare be paying for heart transplants for the estimated 15,000 to 50,000 persons a year who could potentially benefit from the procedure? For that matter, assuming enough organs could be made available, should the program provide liver transplants for the more than 9000 persons who might benefit from that operation? To answer intelligently we have to consider what we know about the potential benefit, and cost, of these procedures at the present time and in the future.

Despite the availability of numerous, voluminous reports and studies, it is difficult, if not impossible, to assess the real success or failure of today's heart and liver transplantation efforts. According to the Office of Transplantation of the U.S. Public Health Service, the one-year survival rate for heart transplant patients is about 80 percent, while liver transplant patients have about a 65-percent chance of surviving the first year. The government estimates the cost of a heart transplant—the transplant and initial hospitalization alone—at $57,000 to $110,000, while a liver transplant is estimated to cost between $135,000 and $238,000. But the government pamphlet that contains these estimates, *Questions and Answers on Organ Transplantation,* then notes that "many variables account for the range of cost in transplantation procedures, i.e., lack of uniformity in reporting component costs, complications, medication regimen, method of reporting or non-reporting payment of surgeons (salary, fee, no charge), graft rejection, readmissions, infections, geography." Which is to say that the Office of Organ Transplantation of the Health Resources Administration of the Public Health Service of the U.S. Department of Health and Human Services has only the vaguest idea what a heart or liver transplant costs. Given how far off the mark federal health officials were in estimating the cost of a kidney dialysis and transplantation program, it is probably safe to assume that, at a minimum, a heart transplant produces bills of at least $150,000 in the first year, while the cost of a liver transplant is at least $250,000. Multiply those costs times the 8500 persons the government estimates could benefit from liver transplants, and the 15,000 it says need heart transplants, and you are staring at a $4,375,000,000 medical bill—and that's for one year!

If heart- and liver-transplant patients could be expected to live out a normal life span, it would be possible to argue that paying $4.375 billion a year for transplants would be cheaper than the long-term costs of treating and hospitalizing these individuals for their disease and losing them from the work force. As Dr. Felix Rapaport, director of transplant services at the State University of New York at Stony Brook and a leader in kidney transplantation since the early 1960s, says, "Humans are the only society in the entire animal kingdom which actually provides ways and means to protect the weak and sickly. Medically, this is a tremendous part of our overall mission. I suspect that if we were to look at this only in cold dollars and cents and turn our back upon medical progress, we will gradually revert back to our roots which we have tried to escape."

Kidney transplants are clearly therapeutic procedures worth the investment being made in them. But how do we determine if heart and liver transplants do indeed represent medical progress, given the dearth of reliable statistics? Not only is there no central source of uniformly gathered and analyzed data, but different transplant centers have different criteria for selecting transplant candidates. Stanford Medical Center, for instance, the nation's premier heart transplant center, is extemely careful in the way in which it screens patients, accepting only those patients who are the "healthiest" and most likely to gain long-term benefits from the operation. However, centers just entering the business are far more likely to accept much sicker patients because their surgeons need to build up their experience in performing transplants and providing the necessary aftercare; those centers therefore will have much poorer survival rates. Is it fair to compare the statistics from an established, top-of-the-line program, such as Stanford's, with those of a start-up program? Probably not. However, the center with the poorer survival rate provides a more accurate picture of what the results of a government-funded, universally available transplant effort would look like.

There are other factors that further cloud the statistical picture. The first is the development of cylosporine, the staggeringly expensive drug that certainly appears to be improving long-term graft survival. But whether it will improve patient survival is another story. That may seem like a contradiction, but as we saw in the case of Philip Koerner, cylosporine is a highly toxic drug that knocks out a patient's immune system so that it is far less likely to successfully reject a foreign organ. But the system that cannot reject an organ is also less likely to succeed at fighting off a microorganism, and it is no exaggeration to say that patients on cylosporine are suffering from iatrogenic (physician-induced) AIDS. In fact, what initially alerted physicians to the existence of AIDS was that otherwise healthy young men were dying of usually benign infections that in the past had killed only those born with defective immune systems or organ transplant patients taking immunosuppressive drugs. So while cylosporine and similar drugs extend the survival time of transplanted organs, we may find over time that they are ultimately killing the organ recipients. During the Vietnam War this type of phenomenon was referred to as "destroying the village in order to save it."

The second factor that muddies the statistical picture is what might be called "bake sale" financing. Because few, if any, centers other than Hershey are willing to say that they accept heart transplantation patients who cannot produce an insurance policy that guarantees payment, or else cannot deposit $100,000 upfront (and the same thing holds true for most liver transplant programs), those patients receiving the operations tend to be those who can raise the money. This means that if a person has a great deal of money, or is well enough loved in the home community to sell $100,000 worth of cakes, cookies, raffle and dance tickets, or is personally appealing enough—an infant or young child, for instance—to receive regional or national media attention, he ends up on the recipient list. So the survival statistics are further confounded by this selection process that has nothing to do with the patient's medical need.

The next variable is that almost all liver transplant recipients are children. It is easy to argue, on ethical, societal and financial grounds that this makes sense. After all, if the transplant succeeds you have saved a person at the beginning of life, who can then grow up and become a functioning member of society. However, the rate at which these children survive the procedure tells us nothing about what the outcome would be for the fifty-five-year-old alcoholic who is likely to be the prime recipient of liver transplantation in a government-funded universal transplant program.

The final major factor that confuses not only the statisical picture but the whole question of organ tranplantation is the shortage of available organs. Although more than 70 percent of Americans believe in the concept of organ donation, they let someone else do the donating, for only 14 percent of those who approve donation carry donor cards.

While many persons, including Arthur Caplan, associate director of the Hastings Center, shudder at the thought of buying and selling human organs, Caplan believes a regulated system of doing just that may eventually be instituted as one solution to the organ shortage. "This was basically outlawed by Congress in 1984 in the National Organ Transplantation Act," he said. "But the situation is going to get worse, not better, and maybe this will change. A second option is presumed consent, which is giving doctors the authority to take organs [from a dead patient] when they need them and have people carry a card when they want to stay out of the system. I think it's ethically defensible, but you have to make sure that the cards are found. It only takes one case of somebody donating when they didn't want to to destroy the whole thing. New York and about five other states have laws that allow coroners to take corneas if they see no outright objection."

One of the most novel solutions to the organ shortage was

suggested about a decade ago by psychiatrist and bioethicist Willard Gaylin, who made the Swiftian proposal that society classify the perhaps 5000 individuals in persistent vegetative states as "Neomorts," and keep them alive as organ farms. When a kidney was needed, it would be taken. Need a cornea? Remove an eye. A heart? No problem. A grizzly solution? Of course. But is it any grizzlier than the present system? Is Gaylin's tongue-in-cheek proposal any more morally repugnant than a system that has transplant coordinators hovering around the parents of a child who has just died, asking for the child's organs in order that "some good can come from this awful tragedy"? Is it any grizzlier than a system that had rich Arabs finding their way to the top of a transplant eligibility list at an American hospital simply because they had money?

So, after thirty-one years of kidney transplantation and eighteen years of transplanting human hearts, we still have not worked out a uniform process either to select patients for these procedures or to pay for them. We have not, in fact, even figured out if we should be providing them. As George Annas asks, "Should we be doing these transplants at all? Are these procedures so expensive that until we have some system to ensure that everyone in America has a basic minimum of health care we shouldn't be adding these extremely expensive halfway technologies? It skews the system. One of my colleagues says aptly: 'We have been doing more and more to fewer and fewer people at higher and higher cost for less and less benefit.' We are getting more and more people who are being completely cut out of the system. Thirty-five million Americans do not have insurance. Most are under twenty-four years old. We are doing more and more medicine to people at the later end of life. When you add something," Annas notes, "you take something away. It's a tradeoff system."

What are the tradeoffs involved in the quickly burgeoning

artificial-heart program? As of 1985, the open-minded can only call this initial program a failure. Barney Clark, the Seattle dentist who served as the first human guinea pig for Dr. William DeVries and his team at the University of Utah, was described to and in the media as a pioneer, a brave explorer of medical frontiers who, in the hopes his life would be extended, agreed to be the first human in whom a Jarvik-7 polyurethane and alloy heart would be implanted. But did Clark have the vaguest idea what he was getting into when he made that agreement? While he may not have honestly believed he would ever go home to Seattle, did he think he would spend his "extra" 112 days in the hospital, slowly deteriorating as his physicians helped him from one medical crisis to the next? Could he have had any way to anticipate a second open-heart procedure to replace a broken—untested—valve in the artificial heart? Could he have anticipated such severe and repeated nosebleeds that he required surgery to stop them? Could he, or should his surgeons, have anticipated an incapacitating stroke—caused by a blood clot formed as a direct result of the artificial heart's use—that would leave him little more than a vegetable? Is that what Barney Clark opted for when he agreed to surgery at the University of Utah?

And what of William Schroeder, the "tough," "spunky" former federal employee and union leader who underwent the same procedure, seemed to be recovering beautifully and then suffered a stroke just as Clark had. We were told he was doing better, but then when the shell of a man was brought before television cameras it was painfully obvious he barely seemed to know who or where he was, or what was going on. Then a great todo was made—by hospital officials and the media—over the fact that Schroeder was leaving the hospital and "going home." But "home" was a special apartment, a specially equipped hospital room, really, less than 120 seconds away from the specialists in the hospital across the street. Then Schroeder suffered yet another stroke and was back in the hospital—where he suffered a third, major stroke. Yes, as of the end of 1985 Schroeder had "survived" for more than a year. But the William Schroeder who survived scarcely resembled the William Schroeder whom surgeon DeVries operated on. Is this the kind of survival Schroeder and his family had in mind when he agreed to the implant?

And what of Murray Haydon? As someone callously but quite aptly described the situation when the Humana Heart Institute International announced that an operation to implant a heart in Haydon had gone "perfectly" and he was bouncing right back, it reminded one of the family who has a dying old dog and goes out and buys a new puppy to distract the children from the death of their beloved pet. Not only did Humana attempt to switch media attention from Schroeder to Haydon, but reporters—and Schroeder's family members—were not even told how bad things looked for Schroeder until *after* the fanfare for the success of the Haydon procedure. And look what happened to Haydon: a second surgical procedure and then "life"—dependent upon a respirator. The next patient, Jack Burcham, died only ten days after receiving the artificial heart. DeVries at least finally acknowledged in an interview that the procedure is experimental, rather than therapeutic. But Robert Jarvik, the inventor of the heart, told *Newsday* medical writer David Zinman that he believes stroke is an acceptable complication to the use of an artificial heart. "Life with stroke is better than death and [is] an acceptable quality of life," said the physician-inventor, who himself has never experienced life either with stroke or with his invention.

Whether or not this quest for eternal life is sensible, a case like Baby Fae's is one in which many people believe the physicians involved overstepped the bounds of acceptable human experimentation. In that case, physicians, guided by their faith in a fundamentalist God, implanted the heart of a baby baboon in a dying infant. The baby, born to poor, unmarried, barely educated parents, might have had a chance at life had she been given an experimental but tested operation to correct her defective heart. She might also have had a reasonable shot had she been given a human heart transplant. But she was not offered any of those things. Instead, she became the first infant to undergo an interspecies transplant, a procedure that has neither succeeded nor given any indication of succeeding in adults, and thus physicians had no realistic reason to expect it to succeed in Baby Fae's case. And even if there was a chance the operation might have succeeded, were her parents honestly informed of the risks? Could they have given truly informed consent?

Though this kind of experimentation is rare indeed, since the Baby Fae case there has been still another one: that of Thomas Creighton. Creighton, a thirty-three-year-old mechanic, was dying of heart disease when surgeons at the University of Arizona gave him a heart transplant. All well and good. But the new human heart was rejected, and so the doctors called for an artificial heart—which they were not authorized to implant. Rather than wait an extra two hours for a Jarvik-7, which has at least been extensively tested on animals and has been cleared by the FDA for human implantation, the Tucson surgeons gave Creighton a heart designed by a dentist and, essentially, never tested. (In a discussion of artificial hearts, twelve hours of testing is tantamount to never being tested.) Then, less than twelve hours after Creighton was given the implant, the surgeons removed it and he underwent a second human heart transplant. That operation, like the first, was a failure, and Creighton died forty-six hours after first being placed on the surgical merry-go-round.

The surgeons justified their action by, one, saying that Creighton would have died without the implant, as though patients don't die every day, and two, saying that doctors answer to a higher power than the FDA. The FDA responded to this clear violation of federal regulation by investigating and then failing to take any action against the surgeon involved. In fact, it later gave him place number three on the list of surgeons approved to implant Jarvik-7's. What message does this send to other doctors who want to carry on their own experiments, using the justification that the patient is dying? What may ultimately be even more disturbing is the fact that the surgeon, Jack Copeland, said he will be using the Jarvik-7 as a bridge to human transplantation in cases where a patient needs a human heart transplant but there is no organ available. Copeland said he views the Jarvik-7 as just "another modality" available to save lives—although at the time it had only been used on five patients and had triggered strokes in four of those.

Even if these problems were not arising, if doctors were not becoming more inclined to experiment on helpless, dying patients, if there were no ethical, legal, bureaucratic or even public relations problems here, we are still left with the question of whether we can afford an artificial-heart program that will cost more than the entire gross national product of many semideveloped nations. It is now estimated that anywhere from 10,000 to 60,000 persons would be candidates each year for an artificial heart implant. Assume there are 50,000. And assume the procedure and attendant treatment will cost *only* $100,000 per patient. That's $5 billion (not million) a year for this one medical procedure. In other words, we would be spending more than twice what we are now spending on kidney dialysis and we will be spending it not to give a new life to children or young adults, but to persons on the verge of retirement, individuals who are likely to develop other diseases and complications in a relatively short period.

Assume, for a moment, that such a program makes social, if not financial, sense. After all, the people receiving these hearts have—at least as a group—contributed to society all their lives and it can be easily argued that they are then entitled to society's support in return. However, once they have been given an artifi-

225

cial heart, what happens when that heart gives out? Bioethicist Robert Veatch makes the interesting argument that, while society does not have an obligation to provide an artificial heart in the first place, it *does* have an obligation to replace that heart when it breaks down. And like refrigerators, artificial hearts will give out, probably in five years or less. Assuming that most individuals receive their first artificial heart at age fifty-five and live another twenty years, we could be talking about supplying each individual with not one but *four* artificial hearts. Or we could be talking about spending not $100,000 per patient but $400,000 per patient, or $20 billion a year.

Clearly, then, it is time for a moratorium on the implantation of artificial hearts. This device may eventually prove to be an enormous boon to mankind. It may save 50,000 lives a year. It may be worth the billions that would be required to make it available. But first we should consider the proper place the device might have in the overall treatment of heart disease after it has been sent back to the animal lab for refinement. The most sensible course of action at this time would be for one of the congressional appropriation committees to establish a national organ transplantation commission to examine the current state of organ transplantation, both natural and artificial. Such a commission should examine the medical, ethical and financial questions at the heart of the transplantation efforts and, as society's representative, make the hard choices that must be made. Should such a commission come down against public funding of organ transplantation, it should decide whether transplants should be available at all. And if it decides that transplants should be publicly funded, the commission should decide what programs will be eliminated to provide the billions of dollars needed to finance a universal organ transplantation program. And, finally, Congress must then be willing to act on the commission's recommendations.

VII.
THE END OF LIFE

CHAPTER 13

The Living Death of Nancy Jobes

The view from room 239A of the Lincoln Park Nursing Home is lovely on this crisp, early autumn afternoon in 1985: Red apples still dot the green of an enormous tree in front of the single-story nursing home complex, and beyond that the sunbathed hillsides of maples and oaks are just beginning to give the first hint of the spectacular display of colors they'll be presenting in a few weeks.

Nancy Jobes is lying on her right side on the room's single hospital bed, as she has for five years, her legs drawn up toward her chest. Her arms lie on the white blanket-cover, which accentuates her dropped wrists and upwardly extended first finger joints. A translucent plastic tube about an inch in diameter snakes from an Aridyne 3500 air compressor beside the bed to the tracheostomy connection on Nancy's throat, carrying moisture to her trachea and lungs. By the head of the bed a Flexiflo Enteral Nutrition Pump sends a slow, steady stream of Isocal complete liquid diet down a one-eighth-inch-diameter clear plastic tube that disappears under the bedclothes, through a surgical incision in Nancy's abdomen into her small intestine. Her open mouth, with its oddly overlapping and twisted teeth, assumes different positions, one moment appearing to smile, the next twist-

229

ing into a hideous grimace. Her large brown eyes are open, roving aimlessly, now *seeming* to fix on a piece of furniture, now on a visitor, now on the world beyond the window. She sees none of it, just as she does not hear the loud voice of the newscaster coming from the portable radio the nurses leave playing by the sink. Her husband, John Jobes, gently smooths back Nancy's hair, and then turns his back to her and stares out the window.

"It was March 11, 1980, and Nancy was on her way to work on a kind of wet, snowy morning," John had said, about an hour before. He was sitting with his in-laws, Eleanor and Bob Laird, in the office of attorney Paul Armstrong, explaining why he, Eleanor and Bob had asked Armstrong to help them force the nursing home to disconnect Nancy's feeding tube to end her life. "She hit a patch of ice in Mountain Lakes and she lost control of the car, and another car coming in the other direction hit her broadside. She was taken to Riverside Hospital in Boonton Township [New Jersey]. It was less than a mile from where the accident was. She sat around the hospital quite a while," John said.

"From early in the morning until late in the afternoon," interjected Eleanor.

"The reason they delayed was they discovered she was pregnant," Bob Laird said, "and there was so much going for the protection of the fetus then that they allowed her to stay in pain without giving her primary treatment. As a matter of fact, they withheld X-rays for quite a number of hours."

"I think John called her obstetrician but he doesn't practice at that hospital and it was recommended that she see one associated with that hospital. He was the one who didn't show to see her until five o'clock. I think it was a communication problem," Eleanor said. She sat with her daughter, who was then a month shy of twenty-five, and kept her company all day. "When the obstetrician examined her—she had been in terrible pain—he found out she had internal bleeding and then everybody started scurrying around. They did emergency surgery that evening, quite good surgery."

After discovering the internal bleeding and finally ordering X-rays, the physicians discovered that Nancy was suffering from a crushed pelvis, a torn bowel and a crushed elbow. At that point, Nancy's interests won out over those of her eighteen-week fetus. "We were all in concert," said Bob Laird, a retired, sixty-year-old engineer. "The bone man was there and it was like he was giving a seminar, because her older sister was there, all three of us were there, and her brother, and we emphasized that she was young and healthy and we didn't want her life at risk, she could always have another child."

"After the surgery I remember somebody remarking that her uterus was still intact, so there was a possibility that the fetus was still alive," Eleanor said.

John said that "Nancy had felt movement of the baby prior to the accident. While she was lying in the intensive care unit recovering after the first operation she kept on worrying that she couldn't feel movement. One of the nurses came in with a stethoscope and said she thought she could hear a heartbeat. Nancy didn't admit it to anybody but me, but she knew she didn't feel movement anymore. I kept trying to tell her it was because of the medication, but she was a pretty determined woman, she was a tiger, she knew what was what."

Sadly, it was finally determined that Nancy Jobes was right: Her fetus was dead, probably killed on impact during the accident. So a suction abortion was scheduled for the removal of the fetus. "She was due to go home two days after having this benign procedure," Eleanor recalled. "April second was the date of the removal. She had already had the surgery on her elbow and she had practiced being left-handed. She had done her bathing and fixed her hair. I remember going in and the lady from the insurance company was there trying to convince Nance she should have a home aide when she went home. And she said, 'No! I am going to be fine. I am going to take care of everything.' She was a very determined girl. She just needed this small procedure done. I said to John, 'I will sit with her, it's so simple. You go to work. Don't take any more time from work.' Nancy was concerned about the procedure," Eleanor said. "The day before I spent the whole day with her and we ate an entire box of Girl Scout cookies."

A few days before the procedure, Nancy, who only three weeks earlier had had surgery to repair a shattered pelvis, had insisted that John help her practice walking down a flight of stairs. But even with all her determination, the confinement was getting to Nancy, John said, recalling that, "the spring flowers were coming up and we were walking down the hospital hall in the warm spring sunshine and she said, 'I want to go home.' "

The morning of the "simple procedure" to remove the dead fetus, Eleanor convinced her son-in-law to go to his machinist's job as she planned on spending the day with Nancy. "They had sedated her and when it was time for her to go down I sat in the room with my sewing. I was even going to go out and get some groceries. And then I heard a code 18 and I heard a nurse run, and I thought, 'Something has gone wrong. What shall you do?' I remember sitting and thinking, 'This is like soap opera. You can't go down, they won't let you in the OR.' So I sat and waited until the nurse came and said the doctor wanted to see me downstairs. They took me down in the freight elevator. I remember thinking specifically that 'This is just like soap opera, this doesn't happen.' The doctor said that he had just started to remove the fetus and her [Nancy's] heart stopped, but they hadn't noticed anything until her skin had mottled" from lack of oxygen.

"The presiding anesthetist was interested in this procedure," Bob said, "so he was standing at her feet and the nurse anesthetist actually administered the anesthesia."

"The anesthesiologist came to the little waiting room where I was and I remember him saying, 'I didn't do it, I didn't do it,' "

232

Eleanor said, who added that someone called John "to tell him the 'simple procedure' didn't work. I remember the doctor coming over and telling me that they got her heart started again and they had her on a respirator."

The hospital called in a neurologist to examine Nancy and, in what would be the first of many parallels between the story of Nancy Jobes and that of Karen Ann Quinlan, the neurologist turned out to be Dr. Robert Morse, who had cared for Quinlan. "He said there would be a forty-eight-hour period. If she was going to come out of it it would be in the next forty-eight hours and there were no guarantees as to the extent of the damage," Eleanor said. "He told us in parable form that it would be better that she die. We weren't ready to accept that. With all her youth and her friends and our other children, there was a lot of hope. So we probably didn't hear exactly what he said. There was never any talk about letting her die at that point. It was full speed ahead with equipment and whatever and we were supportive of that at that point. I remember going in, I think it was the second day, and her eyes finally opened and I thought there was recognition. I guess I thought, 'Oh boy! Everything's going to be all right.' From that point on it was a very, very slow realization that nothing was going to come of it." Nancy was dependent upon a respirator to breathe at that point, Eleanor said, but eventually Dr. Arshad Javed, the same respiratory specialist who had cared for Karen Ann Quinlan, succeeded in weaning her from the machine.

"A lot of Nancy's friends came," John recalled. "I guess maybe [they were inspired by] watching too much TV. They just sat there and talked to her, 'Come on, Nancy, come on, you can fight it.' A lot of very, very good friends."

"Her hands and feet started to turn," Eleanor said. "They have all kinds of equipment to try and keep them straight, but it would just dig into her until they finally had to remove it. She had grown into the position she's in today."

"I don't think we ever really were told there was no hope," John said. "We just had to realize it, in our own way, in our own time."

"We realized as the days, the weeks, the months went by that there was less likelihood of her coming out of it without some kind of impairment," Bob said. Like Joseph Quinlan, Karen Ann's father, Bob Laird was slower than his wife in recognizing, or admitting, that he had lost his daughter.

Eleanor said that she "just started to feel, knowing Nancy, that the kind of recovery, if there was any, was going to have no quality."

John laughed. "She was upset that she was going to have to play tennis with only ninety percent of her elbow. She wouldn't ever want to live a partial life," he said of the lively, athletic young woman he had married in 1976.

A medical laboratory technician, Nancy "used to talk about the children who came in suffering from leukemia. It really tore her up," her father said. "Of our four children, she was the most athletic, even though she was small of stature, five-feet-three. When she was eleven or twelve I asked her what she wanted for her birthday and it was her own baseball glove. In high school she played JV basketball and she was guarding these six-footers—she climbed all over them. She was a really go-getter. . . ."

Extremely shy as a toddler and young girl, Nancy "blossomed when she met this young man, at sixteen, in the toy store where they worked part-time and rode around on the toys when they weren't busy, right?" Eleanor asked John.

"Right. That's when I first asked her out. I rode up on a kiddie car to the register and said, 'Hey, hop in, let's go to the drive-in.' I had just turned seventeen and just gotten my license."

John filed a malpractice suit against the anesthesiology group whose member he and the Lairds held responsible for Nancy's condition, and in 1984 the case was finally settled for about $900,000. After the attorney took his $200,000, John received a cash payment and an annuity that would bring him about $20,000 a year for thirty years, and the Lairds received a cash payment. The no-fault automobile insurance carrier agreed to pay Nancy's medical bills for life, including nursing home charges that by the autumn of 1985 had exceeded $370,000.

But neither cash settlements nor annuities nor medical coverage could do anything to bring back the wife and daughter who had been taken down to the operating room on the morning of April 2, 1980. The money could in no way reconcile John, Eleanor or Robert to the reality of the Nancy who was moved to the nursing home in Lincoln Park, New Jersey.

John initially visited Nancy daily, but then he found himself in room 239A less and less often. "I know that there's nothing I can do over there. And she doesn't know I'm there and all it does is upset me whenever I go. So the way I have to deal with it, for my own well-being and health, is I remember Nancy and all the good points. Every time I go over there, there's nothing I can do. I mean I do go once and a while out of necessity. I was going every other day, the first couple of months, but . . ."

Eleanor continued: "Lincoln Park is about a half-hour trip. We go more frequently. Bob's mother is also a patient at Lincoln Park. She sits by her door frequently and tells us how much Nancy smiles at her and recognizes her. The lady is ninety. She's not senile, but she's very forgetful. She projects much. So Bob and I have gone more frequently, I because she's my infant at this point. But we've cut back to maybe twice a week. We go Sundays after church, that's our usual jaunt, we need to see Mother too." John, Eleanor and Bob all say that, for them, Nancy Jobes died on April 2, 1980. "I think I slowly realized it about two years afterwards," John said. "It took me about two years to realize because of all the well-wishers coming up and saying that something would come on the market, or some new discovery. . . ."

Bob picked up on John's thought. "Occasionally there'd be a story in the newspapers about someone who came out of a coma after four or six months and with therapy would ultimately overcome slurred speech or something like that," he said.

"I think I accepted it a lot sooner because it was easier for me to handle," Eleanor said. "It was easier for me through my religion to think she was with God." An active member of her Presbyterian church, Eleanor said that she gave up hoping a few months after Nancy went into the coma, "even before she went to the nursing home, even though I still talk to her."

"I would say probably it was about the same amount of time for me too," John said, "but I kept having these dreams and I still do. I wake up in a cold sweat. There was one where I was awake and she was standing there in the room and everything was okay and I was apologizing to her for not having faith. It was tough. But Nancy would give me a couple of swift kicks in the rear and say, 'Come on, get on with it.'"

"That's what we're trying to do, get on with it," Eleanor said. "John's a young man and he needs to get on with his life."

Bob Laird came to his decision about Nancy "probably much later than the others, because I still held on to hope for months after she went to the nursing home. But after seeing those dead eyes on a number of occasions it'd confirm it, but then there'd be other occasions when I'd be in there and there'd be a slight noise, or I'd be talking to her, and the eyes would follow and it was almost as though I was talking myself into it, that there was still some hope, still some recognition, but it was spurious. For a long time she's been . . . dead."

Paul Armstrong, who in addition to representing the Quinlans in their historic court battle in the mid-1970s had been involved

236

in more than sixty privately negotiated right-to-die cases, had Nancy examined by several nationally known neurologists, all of whom concluded that she was in a chronic vegetative state and was unable to think or perceive pain or pleasure. However, John said, "It's so hard to accept that she really isn't feeling any pain when your eyes see it in the expression. . . ."

More than a year prior to speaking to Armstrong for the first time, Eleanor Laird began wondering whether it made any sense to continue providing Nancy with nourishment. She said that when she first raised the question with someone, she was advised to be patient and wait until the malpractice suit was settled. "The first time [the nursing home] had any indication [the family might] want feeding stopped was this June when we came back from vacation and Nancy was ready to die," Eleanor said. "She'd lost a lot of weight, and John had tried to stop feeding. John had been in touch with the nursing home because they were looking for permission to put the tube into her small intestine."

"By that time Mom had already met Paul and we wanted to know what we could do, legally, because we don't want to ruin our lives," John said. He, like the Lairds, found it extremely frustrating to have the new tube inserted and Nancy's physical condition improve, only to have to turn around and go to court to have the feeding stopped. But Armstrong believed that if they agreed to having Nancy temporarily transferred to Morristown Memorial Hospital for the insertion of a new tube, they could then take the offense and enter court, fully prepared, to ask that feeding be stopped, rather than be dragged into court fighting a nursing home that was insisting that a procedure was necessary to "save" a patient. So the family members met with nursing home officials and agreed to the transfer to the hospital. "Morally, it's so wrong," Eleanor said, wiping away tears. "Legally, it's correct, but morally it's so wrong to build her up and now she's thriving."

237

John and the Lairds had talked to Nancy's physician at the nursing home about stopping tube-feeding, but had gotten nowhere. "It's understandable. They are doctors and they are supposed to maintain life. You understand their end of it too, but you've got to be a little selfish once in a while," John said.

"The nursing home's position, as I understand it, was going to be, you want to kill Nancy Jobes, fine, but don't do it here. They have no ethics committee," Eleanor said.

"At our meeting with [the doctor] he also threw out something that was disturbing, a case he had heard about in China in which a comatose person had come out of a coma after several years. We pressed him for details to find out where we could read about it, but he couldn't tell us anything," Bob said.

Neither Bob nor Eleanor nor John had any illusions about what they would be asking for in New Jersey Superior Court in Morristown—in the same courthouse and same ceremonial courtroom in which Paul Armstrong had argued the Quinlan case exactly a decade earlier: "Stop feeding her so that she can die," Eleanor said.

"Recognize that she is dead," Nancy's father said. "It's almost analogous to a political prisoner being beaten, and then revived, and then beaten again until they get out what they want. It's horrible in the sense that these resources being expended on her could be used more effectively. More and more the medical people talk about the triage system."

At one point Eleanor consulted with a physician not associated with the nursing home because she wanted to be reassured that withholding feeding from Nancy would not cause Nancy any pain. "I'd been working with a counselor. I thought I was fine. But when I came to thinking that I really would like to see her go, I found that mentally I'm fine but emotionally it means killing my own child. And so I went to [the physician] to be assured she wouldn't feel it. Then I dropped it for about a year until the

238

three of us went back to see him. I needed to set my mind straight. My emotions are still a mess but I needed to set my mind straight that this would be in Nancy's best interest."

"I guess you have to go through something like this to understand that there's no reason to sustain the body when there's nothing else," John said. "It's not helping anybody."

"She is my daughter, my child," Bob Laird said. "I don't want to prolong her suffering, even though medical people say she isn't suffering. But all things must have an ending, 'Time must have a stop,' as I believe Shakespeare once said. We're faced with the mores of society, and you could regard this as murder, or uncaring. And you have the religious aspect of it: One of the ten commandments is 'Thou shall not kill,' it's implicit in our Judeo-Christian ethic. And then finally you have the legal aspect of it, and this is one of the things that's literally fallen through the cracks because it's never been addressed. The fact is that medical ethics is something new and really hasn't been debated in public before, or dramatized, for that matter. And people are bewildered, especially those who have no ken of what's occurring. So what we hope, what we're looking for, what we hope to get are some kind of guidelines where people are absolved of any legal repercussions. The theology of it is way ahead of the legal aspects: the fact that theologians are willing to recognize that if it is their will, people be allowed to go. When you have no proof of it, as in Nancy's case, it gets a little difficult."

Individual members of Nancy's immediate and extended family have dealt quite differently with her situation. "My youngest son-in-law cannot, he just cannot go and see Nancy on the occasions he's been up here," Bob Laird said. "He prefers to remember her as she was."

"Our other children have also drawn back, which is fine," Eleanor said. "Everybody handles it in their own way." Nancy's thirty-two-year-old sister, Elizabeth Ann, who was living in

239

South Carolina, would visit Nancy when visiting New Jersey. But James, Nancy's twenty-seven-year-old brother, and Jean, her twenty-four-year-old sister, avoided visits to the nursing home.

While John Jobes's life was shattered by Nancy's tragedy, it did not come to a complete halt. He busied himself with work, picking up odd jobs after being laid off from his machinist's job, and he slowly began to date again. "These folks here have wanted me to," he said, gesturing toward Eleanor and Bob. "In fact, my mother-in-law set me up." He laughed, and then added, quite seriously, "They want the best for me."

"For the rest of his life John will have some emotional baggage, and it will take an extraordinary woman to put up with it, but we hope that he can resume his life and have children," Bob said. "But he will always be our son-in-law . . . always."

"I tease him that he's going to have two mothers-in-law, poor boy," Eleanor added.

"I've dated," John continued. "I'm thirty-one now and I'd like to have a family. I don't see marriage in the near future anyway. It's just companionship, casual dates. Anytime I think I might have more than that in a relationship, I don't know what it is, maybe it's old school beliefs, or what, but when I took those vows at the altar, that was it, it was 'until death do us part.' But if it came down to I really did fall in love with someone else, and I hope it will happen soon, and Nancy's still in the condition she's in, she hasn't passed bodily away and this hasn't been settled—I would get a divorce. And I don't think anybody would be mad at me."

Eleanor and Bob nodded in agreement. Then Bob said, "John and Nancy did some very wise things," Bob said. "At one point they took a trip around the country."

"My folks said, 'Save your money, buy a house,' " John said. But "a strange thing happened when they visited Lake Tahoe," Eleanor said. "Nancy came back and said, 'When I die, scatter my ashes there.' And that's what we'll do. It sounds strange, but maybe she had a premonition. John and I remembered it when we thought it was going to be the end for Nan . . . what a strange thing for a person her age to think about."

Seeing families go through such a tragedy, one wonders if anything can provide preparation for the ordeal. "It's on-the-job training," Bob said. "The only thing that can prepare you is what kind of childhood you had, the way you were brought up. Your religious mores."

"I don't know where we'd be without our faith," Eleanor said. "And that was late coming in our life. It has been a tremendously growing faith. Our background was Protestant, mild involvement. About ten years ago we joined our present church and began working for the church. Talk about parallels, that's our second home." She was referring to the fact that the parents of Karen Ann Quinlan were tremendously involved in the life of their Roman Catholic parish, and Julia Quinlan, Karen's mother, even worked in the rectory.

Eleanor said she felt compelled to see the problem through to the end, that she couldn't just say to herself, "My daughter is dead," and walk away. "Sometimes I think, 'Wait a minute, this could be an unfair decision. . . . I don't know, I just feel that I want to do right. This is morally right to do in my mind."

But if the court denied the family's request, they could not, they say, attempt to end Nancy's life themselves. "I'm not that courageous. If I was courageous I'd put a pillow over her head. I've also been brought up with a tremendous respect for law and order. This is the law. You do what the law says," Eleanor concluded.

"We've all thought about it," John acknowledged, "but you do what the law says."

"We're not only trying to resolve our own problems, but to make it easier for the next person," Bob said. "I realize that this

241

is a trailblazer, pathfinder kind of thing. I think the thing that influenced me was that book by Gail Sheehy, *Pathfinders.*"

"We need to take a risk," Eleanor said, adding that "we've buried a lot of these thoughts for a long time. I just need to tell you about the beautiful memories we have to hang on to. It was a short life, but a good life. We were blessed to have her. The first time, I guess, when I realized that she was gone was when I first said 'was.' I *had* a child. Once you've said that, then you accept to the core."

CHAPTER 14

Dealing with Dying

The process of dying, the event of death and even the very definition of death have undergone two radical changes in America in this century, changes that have had a major impact on the national consciousness and on the practice of medicine: The deathbed has been moved out of the home and into the hospital; and technology has enabled physicians to interrupt, and therefore extend, the process of dying.

At the turn of the century death was a family-oriented, home-based event. Virtually the only persons who did not die at home were indigent, who might end up in public hospitals, and the institutionalized, who might die where they lived or else in hospital wards. As recently as 1949, almost half of all deaths still occurred at home. That meant most Americans were familiar, if not actually comfortable, with death, having observed closehand the deaths of family members, and dying tended to be a natural, uninterrupted process as a disease followed its natural course.

Today all that has changed: An estimated 80 percent of the almost 2 million persons who will die this year will do so in hospitals and nursing homes, cared for by strangers. What is even more important to our society than the fact that the dying are

243

usually cared for by strangers is the philosophical and professional orientation of those strangers. For rather than being comforters of the dying, they see themselves as preservers of life. Death is the enemy, to be "fought off" at all cost. (It is no mere coincidence that the argot of today's physician is the argot of the battlefield: Treatments are part of the physician's arsenal, a patient is a "victim" of a disease, we are engaged in a "war on cancer.")

When the majority of deaths occurred at home, and pneumonia and influenza were the principal causes of death, death was often viewed as a friend—pneumonia, promising a comparatively graceful passage to the next world, was even referred to as the "old man's friend"—and dying was an inexpensive proposition. If the dying individual was cared for by a physician at all, the only thing the physician could do was to attempt to make the patient comfortable until the end came.

Now, however, with the development and refinement of antibiotics and respirators, influenza and pneumonia have been replaced as leading killers by cancer and heart disease, diseases whose treatment can generate astronomical medical bills. Additionally, with most deaths taking place in institutional settings, where patients are surrounded by the latest life-extending technologies and devices, the process of dying can sometimes be extended to unseemly lengths, at extraordinary expense—for five years at a cost of more than $300,000 in Nancy Jobes's case.

A few short decades ago, you were dead when you were pronounced dead. Everyone—the doctor, the members of your family, the neighbors—everyone knew when death occurred: You were dead when the doctor couldn't hear your heartbeat or see your breath fog a mirror. Or, to put it more simply, you were dead when the doctor said you were dead.

Today, you are still dead when the doctor says you are, for even the more than two-thirds of the states that have legally redefined death in recent years have left it to the attending physician to determine that it has occurred. But watching for two foggy spots on a hand mirror is hardly a way to determine the fact of death in a medical age when an artificial respirator may be keeping the lungs pumping, a dialysis machine may have taken over the function of the kidneys, a surgically implanted tube may be delivering nourishment to the stomach and a left ventricular assist device (LVAD) may be performing the major work of the heart. In such a situation there is always "one more thing" that can be tried to keep the patient alive, always one more experimental treatment, one more antibiotic. Patients who are literally no more than "brain stem preparations," with no cognitive function of any kind, can be kept technically alive for days, weeks and sometimes months or years. And, unfortunately, there is often fear on the part of physicians that if they don't do everything they can conceivably do to keep alive even the most debilitated patient, they will eventually be sued for malpractice by the same relatives of the patient who may be telling them to give up. Physicians may even worry about the possibility of criminal prosecution for "mercy killing," although no physician has ever been convicted of that crime in this country.

For some time the bioethical literature was replete with debates over the fine points of "active" versus "passive" euthanasia. While there are still some ethicists and theologians trying to establish just how many angels can dance on the head of that particular pin, certainly most practitioners realize that the only question is one of semantics, rather than practice. Some ethicists argue that omitting an act, such as resuscitation of a terminally ill patient who has suffered a massive heart attack, is "passive," while committing an act, such as turning off a respirator, is "active" euthanasia and therefore illegal. Certainly the public posture of most physicians is governed by their awareness of these legal and ethical niceties. But if a physician is acknowledged to have the right to stop a course of antibiotics when he sees that his patient's condition fails to improve, cannot another physician turn off a respirator when she sees that her patient is not improving? Who, after all, is playing God, the physician who turns off a respirator and allows the natural process of dying to conclude, or the physician who turns on the respirator and interferes in that natural process?

Physicians have, in any case, been "playing God," with little complaint from the congregation, ever since the first surgeon stepped on a battlefield. The dispensing of military medicine is based on the concept of triage, deciding who can most benefit from treatment and treating those persons first. Thus, the soldier with a minor wound is made to wait while the more severely injured soldier is treated. And rather than waste valuable time and resources on the soldier who is unlikely to ultimately recover and return to battle, he is left to wait—die—in line behind the least severely injured. Most hospital emergency rooms have either a nurse or a physician on triage duty, deciding who should be seen first and who can wait. The only real difference between the military and civilian systems is that the sickest, most severely injured patient is theoretically seen first in the civilian setting, whether or not their condition looks hopeless.

The arrival of mechanical life-support systems on the medical scene complicated the standard decision-making process, in large part because it made the decisions, and actions, of physicians so clear. With the flick of a switch, the physician could turn on the respirator, or ventilator as it is properly called, to "save" a patient, or turn it off to "kill" her. The enormity of that action was troubling to physicians themselves, so troubling, in fact, that in 1957 a group of anesthesiologists asked Pope Pius XII for guidance on their moral obligation to keep the respirator on or turn it off. The Pope then told them that there was no moral obligation to use this new technology to sustain life where there was no hope of recovery.

But today, anyone visiting a modern intensive care unit can see that that is exactly what is often being done. The sickest patients lie on their beds, literally surrounded by machines. In a typical unit a Bennett MA-1 respirator—the kind used to sustain Karen Ann Quinlan—may stand by the bedside, a length of plastic tubing snaking from the machine across the patient's usually frail chest to either a smaller tube forced down the patient's trachea or a small fitting surgically implanted through the neck, into the trachea. Various colored wires crisscross the bed, leading from the patient's body to machines used to monitor the patient's blood pressure, heart and respiration rates. Not only is the patient often unable to recognize his own children, but the patient's children are sometimes unable to recognize a parent submerged in a sea of tubes and wires. In one particularly telling incident, a man called a newspaper to find out who gave the paper permission to run a picture of his mother hooked up to a respirator and lying on her side in a hospital bed. It turned out that not only wasn't the patient the man's mother, but the "mother" was a man.

Unlike most forms of medical "progress," which cause overnight public sensations but little serious discussion, these changes in the way we die have become the subject of intense, if sporadic, public debate. Because an alert, competent adult has the legally recognized right to refuse medical treatment, even if that refusal will bring about his death, most of the attention to these issues has centered on the question of when life-sustaining care can be withdrawn from those not competent to make decisions for themselves.

For more than a decade, the case of Karen Ann Quinlan served as the focal point of the debate. At the time she became comatose, in April 1975, terms such as "chronic vegetative state," "right to die," "hospice" and "living wills" were unknown to most Americans. In fact, such terms and the issues they raised were so foreign to most persons that it came as a shock when, during the Quinlan trial, Karen's mother testified that her daughter had once said, "Never let them keep me alive by artificial means, Mommy." Who could believe, such a long decade ago, that a twenty-one-year-old woman with only a high school education sat around having such conversations with her mother? Death was a topic to be avoided, not brought up around the Formica kitchen table.

But if the Quinlan case did nothing else, it, along with the work of Elisabeth Kübler-Ross, brought the subjects of dying and death out of the churches, nursing homes and hospitals and into the kitchens, living rooms and bedrooms of America. The "girl in the coma," as the headline writers and television newscasters referred to Quinlan, became a symbol of a growing national debate, for the Quinlan case made countless millions of people aware that circumstances could conspire to make them prisoners of the very technology designed to save them.

Had Karen Ann Quinlan died when her father finally won his legal battle and her respirator was turned off, then the New Jersey Supreme Court's decision in the matter of Karen Ann Quinlan might have become an historical footnote, a matter of intense interest only to legal scholars and those caring for the dying and hopelessly ill. But Karen Quinlan did not die. Instead, she lived in a coma for more than a decade, finally dying on June 11, 1985. Her case remained at the edge of our collective peripheral vision as the media carried occasional stories about her parents' daily visits to her bedside or about the annual bedside mass held on her birthday. The Quinlan case, like no other, held our interest and focused attention on these issues because if a healthy young woman like Karen Ann Quinlan could spend a third of her "life" locked in a fetal position in a chronic vegetative state, weighing as little as sixty-five pounds, then the same thing could happen to any of us.

The day Quinlan finally died, George Annas, professor of

health law at Boston University's schools of medicine and public health and one of the nation's leading experts on health law, was asked what word or phrase came to mind when he heard the name Karen Ann Quinlan. "I don't want to be like," Annas responded without pausing. "The thing the Quinlan case has done for most people is kind of set up a paradigm," Annas said. "People say, 'I don't want to die like Karen Ann Quinlan.' It's a very important thing her case has done. A lot of people write living wills just for that reason. Her tragedy really has helped a lot of people and it's gotten a lot of people to think about things they wouldn't have thought about otherwise—like how they might die and what people might do to keep them alive."

Since the Quinlan case, whenever the issues of patient self-determination, "the right to die with dignity" and euthanasia, or mercy killing, seem to have slipped from the public consciousness, a new case or incident has made the headlines and rekindled the debate. In the Saikewicz case in Massachusetts, officials of Belchertown State Hospital sought to withhold chemotherapy treatments from a sixty-six-year-old, profoundly retarded resident of the institution. The officials contended that the chemotherapy would only extend Joseph Saikewicz's life for a short time and that he would be unable to understand the discomfort and pain to which he was being subjected. A probate judge in Northampton, Massachusetts, ruled that Saikewicz must be treated. The highest state court, however, ruled against treatment but held that such decisions are properly heard in the courts, not settled privately on the back wards of hospitals.

There have been a number of cases in the New York area that have been similar to Quinlan's in that they have, in effect, extended to the hopelessly ill, incompetent patient the same right to refuse treatment—albeit through a guardian or relative—held by the competent patient, or they have restated that traditional right of the competent patient to refuse life-sustaining medical care.

B. D. COLEN

In the Brother Fox case, the court of appeals—New York's highest tribunal—upheld a lower court ruling that a comatose, elderly cleric could be removed from the respirator that was sustaining his life. The court held that its judgment could be substituted for that of the comatose Brother Fox, ruling as it believed he himself would want the case decided. In the case of Peter Cinque, a court granted a popular teacher whose health was quickly deteriorating the right to stop the kidney dialysis treatment he needed to maintain his life. While neither this case nor the Quinlan case involved an enunciated "right to die," the Cinque court upheld the principle of the patient's right to self-determination, holding that Cinque, who was mentally competent, could not be forced to undergo life-sustaining treatment.

Perhaps the most publicized but least meaningful case since Quinlan was Elizabeth Bouvia's unsuccessful fight for death. When she was twenty-six, the quadriplegic cerebral palsy victim went to court to force a Riverside, California, hospital to aid her in starving to death. A superior court panel denied her request without comment, presumably because she was asking a hospital to aid her suicide. Despite the tremendous amount of media attention engendered by Bouvia, this case really had little to do with the major issues central to the care of the dying. Bouvia was not asking for the right to reject heroic medical intervention. She was not even asking, as a dying patient, that "ordinary" care, such as feeding and antibiotic treatment, be withheld. For she was not dying. Rather, she was asking to remain in the hospital for the express purpose of being kept comfortable while she ended her life by starvation.

While the Bouvia case did little but keep a number of attorneys and reporters busy, the little-noticed case of Selma Saunders, a seventy-year-old, terminally ill woman from Oceanside, New York, may well have carried the Quinlan doctrine several steps farther. Saunders, who was suffering from both lung

250

cancer and emphysema, wanted assurance before entering a hospital, presumably for the last time, that her wishes would be honored and she would be disconnected from life-support systems if she was deemed at some future time to be irreversibly comatose. She had filled out a living will, expressing these wishes, but was told by the hospital that it would not be bound by her wishes. But Justice Bernard McCaffery ruled that "the right of a terminally ill competent adult to discontinue extraordinary treatment is well established. . . . This court finds that this right to refuse or discontinue extraordinary medical treatment is not lost when and if they suffer irreversible brain damage, become comatose, and are no longer able to personally express their wishes. . . . Since incompetent persons may not exercise this right while they are incompetent, there must be provided a means by which this right may be exercised on their behalf, otherwise it will be lost." While McCaffery did not declare Saunders's living will legally binding as such, he did hold that it had the same status as "an informed medical consent statement authorizing the refusal" of medical treatment. (Of the more than two dozen states that have legally recognized the living will, a statement in which a person, while in good health, declares his wishes concerning the use of life-sustaining treatment should he ever become incapacitated, only in the District of Columbia is the living will legally binding upon physicians attending the will's maker.) But more important than whether McCaffery did or did not make living wills legally binding, he held that physicians honoring Saunders's advance refusal of treatment could not later be held liable by members of the woman's family who might disagree with her decision and attempt to sue the doctors for honoring it.

While few families have suffered through the kind of agony that was the Quinlan family's life for a decade, literally millions of Americans have had to, or will have to, make hard choices regarding treatment of terminally ill relatives, or its withdrawal.

251

B. D. COLEN

Such decisions may seem clear-cut when viewed from afar, but they are rarely simple for those involved.

Physicians weighing family requests must first of all consider what is best for the patient, what the patient's quality of life will be if therapy is continued, and whether the patient, rather than the physician or the family, would consider that quality of life acceptable. Physicians must consider the possibility that family members seeking the withdrawal of life support have something to gain by the patient's immediate death. And, unfortunately, physicians must sometimes consider what the bills generated by a patient's lingering death will mean to the survivors. As was noted in the introduction to this book, most Americans tend to look the other way when decisions are made regarding the dollar value of human lives: We don't always insist that cars be made safer, that factory emissions be made cleaner or that coal mines be made safer because each of those things would cost money. Instead, we passively accept the loss of lives those savings entail. Ironically, however, we have often been more willing at least to consider such equations when the setting for that consideration has been a hospital or a physician's office.

What middle-aged or older physician can honestly say he never considered the expense to the family of operating on a senile eighty-year-old patient? And is it unusual for the middle-aged children of elderly patients with Alzheimer's disease to wonder what is accomplished by spending $30,000, $40,000 or more than $50,000 a year for the nursing home care of a father who can no longer recognize his children? Ethicists and moral theologians have long considered such questions. In fact, the often-used term "extraordinary means" encompasses expenses that would create an "extraordinary" burden to a patient or a patient's family. According to leading American Catholic bioethicists, such as the Rev. Richard McCormick, S. J., the Catholic Church, which since the Middle Ages has held that there is no moral obligation to use extraordinary means to sustain life, includes financial burden in the definition of "extraordinary." As McCormick has explained it, if a family would have to go bankrupt to pay for care to keep a family member alive, and the other members of the family would suffer undue hardship because of that, such expenditures would be extraordinary and would not be morally obligatory.

The purchase of extra days or weeks of life for the terminally ill carries a high price tag. An astounding 28 percent of the budget of the Medicare program for the elderly is spent on the last year of life of the 5 percent of Medicare patients who die in a given year. That amounted to no less than $17 billion in 1982—and doesn't include state or private funds. The sum is more than three times what the federal government spent on medical research. As Richard McCormick has pointed out, "We're spending too much money on people in the last years of their lives." And because most deaths now occur in the hospital, and the American population is aging, more and more hospital intensive care beds are being devoted to extending the dying process of the terminally ill elderly, rather than curing acutely ill individuals who might be expected to recover.

For example, at North Shore University Hospital in Manhasset, New York, an eighty-one-year-old man was admitted to the cardiac intensive care unit in March 1981 and remained there until he died in August of that year. His five-month stay in a unit designed to care for patients for about ten days cost $142,920.50, and today would cost well over $200,000. A seventy-nine-year-old woman admitted to the same unit on November 19, 1983, remained there until her death the following March 22. Her bill exceeded $120,000.

According to Dr. Peter Reiser, director of medical and cardiac intensive care at North Shore, at any given time up to about 15 percent of the intensive care beds—as many as six or seven at once—are taken up by elderly patients who cannot be weaned from respirators and cannot be sent to any other institution. These patients, said Reiser, are "trapped in ICUs."

"We're on very shaky ground if we were to terminate ventilator [respirator] support without a court order," said the physician, explaining that it is the policy at his hospital to continue respirator support unless and until a court order is obtained.

This does not mean, however, that Reiser and his colleagues go all out to maintain all life at all cost. Rather than actively turn off the respirator, Reiser said he engages in a "form of benign neglect: You cannot institute a form of therapy." He cited an example involving a patient with an infection: "You get the cultures back and the cultures come back positive. You're under legal and moral obligation to treat the infection for ten to fourteen days. At the end of that period we're not obligated to get more cultures. We'll treat vigorously for whatever it takes to give the patient a chance." But after that, he said, the vigor diminishes. If it doesn't, Reiser warns, he can foresee a day in this generation when patients will be refused admission to ICUs because they may end up using more than their share of available resources.

In an earlier day, when the national checking account seemed bottomless, we didn't need to worry about the expense of maintaining a patient in a vegetative life. And even a few years ago, when Medicare paid for care on the basis of days of hospitalization and services rendered, hospitals and physicians didn't have to give much thought to the cost of the care they were providing a given patient—other than making sure that that patient had health insurance.

Today, with the advent of the DRG (Diagnostic-Related Grouping) system of Medicare reimbursement, a hospital can ill afford to keep a heart attack patient in an ICU for three months. Under the DRG system, Medicare reimburses a flat payment for a given diagnosis. Thus, a hospital might be paid $10,000 for caring for a heart attack patient because Medicare had determined that, on average, heart attack patients spend five days in the coronary care unit at $1000 a day and another five days in a less expensive room. Those charges, plus other hospital costs, might average $10,000. A hospital that could get the patient in and out of the CCU in three days, rather than the usual five, and out of the hospital in another four days would stand to make money under the DRG system. But if, as in the case of the woman at North Shore who was hospitalized for months beyond the usual stay, the patient ran up an astronomical bill, the hospital would have to take a loss. Obviously, such a system will make hospitals think twice before they take on difficult cases. It may, in fact, eventually force some hospitals to drop some of their services.

But do the patients who are "benefiting" from these expensive technologies and services view them as a benefit? Not always. In a study published in 1983 in the *New England Journal of Medicine*, a group of health-cost experts and bioethicists concluded that society has not yet reached the point where it cannot afford what it is spending on the terminally ill. But most experts agree there are hard choices ahead in this area. As physicians have become increasingly skilled at maintaining the last semblances of life, they have had to deal with increasing frequency with the question of whether and when they should refrain from using those skills. And while court cases involving decisions to turn off life-sustaining respirators—actively "pulling the plug"—make for media drama, a group of researchers found that such decisions are commonplace in the nation's hospital intensive care units. And poll after poll has found that the public, rather than suing doctors who turn off life-sustaining respirators, overwhelmingly support the concept of ending care in hopeless cases.

The study group, headed by Dr. Jack Zimmerman, director of

255

the intensive care unit at George Washington University Medical Center surveyed the practices in twenty ICUs in fourteen hospitals across the country, ICUs that served 4700 patients in 1982. "Do Not Resuscitate" (DNR) orders were written for 417, or 5.6 percent, of those patients. According to the survey, 54 percent of those 417 patients were over sixty-five and 39 percent were in severely failing health. And 94 percent of those for whom DNR orders were written died during that hospital stay, with 74 percent dying in the ICU.

In theory, a "No Code," or "Do Not Resuscitate," order written for a patient suggests that the physician caring for the patient has decided that the patient's best interests would not be served by attempting to restart the heart, should it fail, or by restoring breathing. But Zimmerman believes his survey shows "No Codes" may mean more than that. Examining the 199 No Code cases in thirteen institutions other than George Washington, the Zimmerman group found that "eighty-seven percent were in the ICU less than three days."

In an interview shortly after the study was published in *Critical Care Medicine* in March 1984, Zimmerman said: "Something happened there all of a sudden, and deciding to not do something had something to do with it." He added that "when a 'No Code,' a Do Not Resuscitate, order is written, the average time to either death or discharge from the ICU is less than two days, and we think that implies that many DNR decisions involve withholding or withdrawing life support." In fact, he said, the study indicates that "when DNR orders are written they are accompanied by decisions to withdraw support about forty percent of the time."

At George Washington, said Zimmerman, decisions are frequently made to withdraw respirator support from patients in the No Code group. Such decisions are made, he said, "for a number of reasons." One reason is that the patient simply has not responded and is unlikely to respond to further treatment. However, he stressed, "It is very important to recognize that these decisions are ones that are made jointly between physicians and patients or, more commonly, families."

We may worry that physicians and family members may not always opt for resuscitation when a patient might want it. However, a study published in the April 26, 1984, issue of the *New England Journal of Medicine* found that eight of the twenty-four mentally competent, chronically ill patients who were resuscitated in 1981 while at Boston's Beth Israel Hospital wished they had been allowed to die. Drs. Susanna E. Bedell and Thomas L. Debanco, who conducted the study, wrote, "Our study suggests that many patients may know what they want and welcome the chance to make their own contributions to this difficult debate." While the authors noted that the patients had varying reasons for wishing they had not been resuscitated, they "were focused primarily on their discontent with a life-style limited by chronic illness and their fear of further suffering at the time of [cardiac] arrest and resuscitation."

Although Zimmerman practices in the one U.S. jurisdiction, the District of Columbia, in which living wills are legally binding upon physicians, he says it is rare to encounter such a document. Rather, he said, decisions to withhold or withdraw life-extending care follow an assessment that "the patient has not responded and is unlikely to respond to further treatment." While Hastings Center Director Daniel Callahan believes the publicity attendant to the Quinlan case and similar cases has publicized the issue of withdrawing care and thus made it more difficult for physicians to turn off respirators, Zimmerman believes the opposite. "I find that in my own practice, if anything, because these issues are much more in the public eye, they have become easier to deal with. I think that patients and families talk about these things a lot more now than they did when the Quinlan case came up, that while there's a tremendous variation in physician practices, that dialogue leads to a more frank discussion of the issues at hand and very often leads to the withdrawal of life support."

Decision making in this area often becomes muddied when younger physicians, particularly house staff, are involved, said Dr. Ronald Bishop, a professor of medicine and cancer specialist who runs the medical ethics program at the University of Michigan. "This is a situation that I don't think is well understood by much of the house staff because they think they are the prime decision makers. My own viewpoint," said Bishop, who has been practicing medicine for more than three decades, "is that in the ideal situation the patient should be making the decision, either by committing himself by a living will or discussing the situation with his family. If he's competent, we can discuss it with him. I do feel No Code decisions should be reached by a meeting of the minds between staff and family and others involved. If there's resistance, and there's truly a matter of scarce resources, then the physician does have to make a decision, but we don't have to make that decision very often."

Bishop could recall, however, "a situation we had a lot of fun with here involving a patient with a neurological disease that was going toward its inevitable termination. The patient had had recurrent pulmonary infections and was brought into the ICU on the pulmonary service," Bishop said. "The patient was, in many respects, in a vegetative state, and the family wanted everything done for the patient. Apparently, everything was being done for the patient at home, although she was nonresponsive except to pain. So there came a conflict between the treatment team on the ward and the family because the family thought she should be on positive Code status and the house staff thought she should be a No Code. They did give her antibiotics and cured her pneumonia and she was discharged once again, but the staff said the only way she'd be readmitted was on a No Code status, and I think they let the family know that. It could be argued she could go to another hospital."

At the time, Bishop was holding monthly ethics seminars at his home, and on the night that case was discussed the house was "overflowing with people who wanted to discuss the case."

While decisions to turn off respirators or actively withdraw life support are frequently not openly discussed, or are even denied, many hospitals have become very open about their No Code policies. A DNR order is the result of a decision not to call the "Code Blue" (cardiac resuscitation), team when a terminally ill patient suffers a heart attack, or not to place such a patient on a respirator should he stop breathing.

At the University of Michigan Hospital, such No Code orders are formally entered into the patient's chart, according to Edward Goldman, the hospital's attorney. "It must be a written order on the chart or the patient is considered a full code," which means staff members will go all out to sustain life, Goldman said. The question of whether to issue a No Code order is "discussed with the patient if the patient's competent," Goldman said, "or discussed with the family if the patient can't understand." Goldman said "the idea" of writing the order on the chart is to make sure that the hospital does "not put decision making in an inappropriate place, in other words, not have the nurses try to decide what to do." The procedure was put in place by the hospital's executive committee on clinical affairs and is appropriate, he said. "Doctors," Goldman said, "have to make those decisions."

But are No Code orders legal?

"The courts make a distinction between action and reaction," Goldman said. "No Code has been seen as a decision not to start something, rather than as a decision to stop." There are no relevant court precedents in Michigan, Goldman said in early 1984, adding: "I would hope the courts would say that if you're following informed-consent notions, and if you're doing the No Code because the underlying condition of the patient is irreversible, untreatable, that's okay."

Because of the nonexistent state of the law on No Codes in

most jurisdictions, hospital policies vary on whether or not to record No Code orders. At North Shore on Long Island, No Code orders are indeed issued but are not put in writing, as they are at Michigan and at George Washington. "I don't think we write No Code orders here," said Richard H. Beresford, a physician and attorney who serves as chairman of neurology at North Shore and teaches law and medicine at Cornell University in Ithaca. "Many people don't write the order, but there is an understanding. . . . It is part of medical practice not to provide certain types of care" for certain types of patients, he said. The lack of law on the No Code issue creates uncertainty on the part of physicians, Beresford continued, "which means you're very careful what you do. You worry about it, you worry about it, you worry about it," he said. "And then you do something."

In March 1984, staid and highly respected Memorial Sloan-Kettering Cancer Center in New York City was the object of tabloid headlines such as "Prosecutor Demands Hospital Action: 'BAN SECRET DEATH LISTS,' " not because it kept its No Code list secret but because it was open about its coding. In fact, the hospital was using blackboards in doctors' lounges to record No Code orders. Patients at Sloan-Kettering were listed on the blackboards with letters A, B, C or D next to their names. The A patients were those diagnosed as having an excellent chance of recovery, or whose disease had not then been diagnosed, and everything was done for them. The B patients had cancer but were thought to have a chance of recovering, and they, too, would be resuscitated. The C patients were diagnosed as terminally ill and would only be made comfortable, rather than being coded. The D patients were those believed to be beyond benefiting from anything the physicians could do for them. Sloan-Kettering officials said that the "secret death lists" were discussed with both patients and families.

Since that time, both New York State Health Commissioner

David Axelrod, M.D., and a commission appointed by governor Mario M. Cuomo to study bioethical issues have recommended that any No Code orders be fully discussed with patients and/or family members and be made a part of the permanent medical record.

Even more central than the question of coding to the ongoing debate over whether or when to withdraw life-sustaining treatments have been two terms, concepts really: "ordinary" versus "extraordinary" care, and "active" versus "passive" euthanasia. While it is generally recognized that health care professionals have a duty to provide ordinary care to even a terminally ill patient hours away from death, many persons would argue there is no such obligation to provide extraordinary, or "heroic," care. But in an age in which terms such as "CAT scan" have entered the vocabulary of even the most medically unsophisticated, what is extraordinary? Is it extraordinary to use a respirator on a patient in an intensive care unit? Those who argue that life must always be preserved at all costs would argue not. On the other hand, many respected physicians would argue, along with the husband and parents of Nancy Jobes, that it is extraordinary to provide something as basic as nourishment to a comatose patient with no chance of recovery.

Feeding has, in fact, become the "respirator" of the 1980s. Now that courts in several states have acknowledged that there may come a time when an "extraordinary" life-sustaining treatment, such as the use of a respirator, may be withdrawn, the current question is whether it is ever right to stop providing a patient with care as basic as feeding. The New Jersey Supreme Court, which paved the way for other states in the Quinlan case, may have done the same thing in the case of Claire Conroy. In that case the court held that life-sustaining feeding could be ended for the eighty-four-year-old semicomatose woman who suffered from heart disease, diabetes, a gangrenous left leg and

261

other medical conditions. Writing for the majority in the court's six-to-one decision, Associate Justice Sidney M. Schreiber, who had been a member of the Quinlan court almost exactly a decade earlier, held that "analytically, artificial feeding by means of a nasogastric tube or intravenous infusion can be seen as equivalent to artificial breathing by means of a respirator. Both prolong life through mechanical means when the body is no longer able to perform a vital function on its own."

Boston University's George Annas said he doesn't see a great deal of difference between the Quinlan and Conroy decisions, or, for that matter, between those cases and the Jobes case in that all three cases hinge on "the right of competent people to refuse anything. The rights of incompetent patients have to be derived from the rights they have if they're competent. If you're competent, you can refuse feeding. I really don't think you can separate these things," Annas said. "Part of the question is the treatment and part of the question is the prognosis: What am I going to be like? What things am I going to be able to do and what things am I not going to be able to do?"

A. J. Levinson, executive director of the group Concern for Dying, said at the time of Karen Ann Quinlan's death that "the issues have gotten well beyond Karen Quinlan and the removal of the respirator to the question of whether alimentation can be removed—whether one can refuse in advance to have one's body invaded by artificial plastic tubing through which nutrition is pushed." Isn't it somewhat misleading to refer to feeding, which we all understand, as alimentation, which has such a foreign, clinical, sound to it? "There is a connotation to the word 'feeding' that includes comfort, care, love and concern, all the emotions that are involved in love. That is feeding," she replied, "and the word 'feeding' carries all those emotional, contextual factors. My concern is that the provision of vitamins, minerals and electrolytes is not feeding: Feeding is a ham sandwich, a milkshake or ginger ale."

The Rev. John Connery, S.J., does not worry about the focus of the discussion moving from the use of respirators to the question of feeding. Rather, the professor emeritus at Loyola University in Chicago, who served as an adviser to the Quinlan family in their historic court battle, worries that the debate is changing in more insidious ways. "In those days," said Connery, referring to the mid-1970s, "the focus was on treatment, on the morality of removing life-sustaining treatment. We used to rely on the distinction between ordinary and extraordinary means to preserve life. Today, the tendency is to move away from determining the norm of the quality of the means, or treatment, and to shift it over to discussing the quality of life, what lives one should preserve and what lives one is obligated to preserve. This is a precarious approach to the whole question," said John Connery. "Some people are in favor of making quality-of-life decisions, but we have no norms, no way to draw lines in regard to quality of life. What quality of life is above the standard, and what quality of life is below?"

Moral theologians like John Connery do not want us asking, much less answering, such questions. But the time has long since passed when we can avoid dealing with these issues, for the basic issue of quality of life lies at the heart of all the hard choices discussed in this book: If we choose to eliminate genetic defects we are making a statement about the quality of life of those now living with such defects; if we hold to the position that human embryos have "rights" and cannot be experimented upon, then we have to seriously reconsider our societal decision to allow them to be aborted simply because they interfere with a woman's quality of life; when we argue for or against the right of parents and physicians to withdraw care from hopelessly ill or defective newborns, we are engaging in a debate over quality of life. We can no longer afford to hide behind the rationale that we must save all life at any cost. We can no longer afford to do so. If we are going to save every "life," regardless of the quality of that life,

263

then the federal government must pay the $300,000 bill for a liver transplant and care of a sixty-year-old alcoholic, as well as for a two-year-old child. Applying the same logic, if we provide one artificial heart transplant to an individual, then we are going to have to provide five.

Some experts in the fields of health care, bioethics and economics have concluded that we are a long way from having to make the financial hard choices engendered by modern medical technology. Would that they were right. But we can no longer base health care decisions in the hope that Congress will choose to fund liver transplants rather than a B-1 bomber. We have seen enough gutting of social programs in the past four years to know that that kind of one-for-one tradeoff does not occur. A decision to build fewer bombers translates into a commitment to fund Star Wars research, not a commitment to fund Medicare heart transplants.

No, these medical and bioethical hard choices are not the stuff of some futuristic nightmare: They are part of our present reality. They are, in fact, being made on a daily basis. But they are not being made by us or by our legislators. They are being made by bureaucrats in the federal Office of Management and Budget. The decisions are being made in the name of budgetary planning and constraint, but they amount to social planning and engineering as surely as if they were the result of the carefully considered work of committees of ethicists and philosophers. Unless we are happy having these hard choices made for us on a purely financial basis by the same sorts of managers who would declare ketchup a vegetable in a school lunch, we must insist that making these choices become part of our national political debate.

Acknowledgments

There are a number of persons who, in one way or another, made the writing of this book possible. First among these is Jamie Talan, whose research and interviewing for four of the chapters proved invaluable. Kenneth Paul, *Newsday* specialists' editor—and a friend—read the manuscript at various stages of its development and made numerous important suggestions. Thanks to Joan Sanger, my editor at Putnam, who maintained faith in this project even when mine wavered and provided excellent editing. My wife, Sara, and children, Benjamin, Alicia and Nicholas, were patient and understanding through my periods of absence, both physical and mental, and for that I am most grateful. And, finally, special thanks to the literally dozens of persons who over the course of the past decade have allowed me into their lives and laid bare their souls under the most trying of circumstances. Without them I could not have begun, let alone finished this book. For their dilemmas are ultimately what this book is all about.

Index